ANDREW'
LIVING WITH P.....

By Brenda Prentice

'One million people commit suicide every year'
The World Health Organization

Brenda Prentice

Published by
Chipmunkapublishing
PO Box 6872
Brentwood
Essex CM13 1ZT
United Kingdom

http://www.chipmunkapublishing.com

Edited by Kimberley Bishop

Cover photo by April Prentice.

'*he remains what he has always been, tee-total*'

ANDREW'S STORY

Preface

Oh no! That feeling, the usual discomfort that I
permanently suffer has just altered ever so
slightly. I feel the blood rush to my face and that
horrible realisation, that paranoia. My mood drops
like a leaden weight and my mind switches so all
that I can now think of is getting home quickly.

I just received the first signal from my body that I
am about to have another attack of Pancreatitis. It
could be a false alarm; God knows I have them
almost every day lately. I just know by the
constant discomfort, others may call it pain but I
term it as discomfort, pain is something else that I
have, it is starting to burn. It will eventually be a
nagging burning pain situated on the upper right of
the abdomen, which will gradually increase and
then radiate across my chest and around to my
lower back. However, before we get there I will
have a lot more to get through first. "Here we go."
I am now feeling queasy and break out into a light
cold sweat. I feel the urgent need for bowel
movement but know that if I sat on the lavatory
nothing will happen. Now I am burping, bringing
up small amounts of acidic bile and have rampant
heartburn. While I quickly clear my desk, a
colleague looks across at me and instantly knows
by the grey hue of my face and sweaty brow that I
am beginning an attack. They have seen this
before at my office. Previously someone used to

drive me the twenty three miles home while I would throw up into a bag throughout the journey but nowadays I prefer to get home under my own steam (a mixture of retaining a small amount of dignity and preventing the problem of having to leave my car at work for however long). I have since learnt how to throw up and drive at the same time. Speed is of the essence though I am also aware that if I react quickly when I get the signals I can often make it home before the vomiting really kicks in.

I manage to pull up on my drive, throw open the car door and projectile vomit across the lawn. I haven't managed to get my seat belt off in time and manage to splash vomit all over me and the car door, interior of course. As I get out of the car I find I can not stand up straight now because of the pain. I walk into the house stooped over and crawl straight up the stairs to the bathroom. I feel slight relief to be home now but that feeling of relief is over very quickly as I start vomiting again. When I have an attack I can see the layers of food come back up in the order that I ate them (often going back days) looking almost the same as it did on the plate. I remain in the bathroom about three quarters of an hour throwing up spending the time contemplating what had triggered this particular attack. Was it something I ate? Was it stress? Had I physically overdone it? I monitor the layers of vomit for clues as to when exactly my wonderful

ANDREW'S STORY

pancreas decided to start eating itself again and my stomach stopped digesting this time. Once the solids are up, I am now only bringing up clear frothy bile. I retire to my bed with a sick bucket and a large bottle of water. That will be me for probably the next forty eight hours or so.

NAUSEA and nauseam, It's not the pain at the moment. My tormentor is nausea, don't get me wrong, the pain is there alright but the nausea just takes over in waves for forty minutes or so and then I will retch and retch until I bring up some more frothy yellowish bile. This is followed by about five minutes of relief from the nausea which allows me to concentrate on the pain for a short time. A deep pain is now in the centre of my body like someone or something has bored a six-inch hole through me and is now honing it out slowly with some kind of cheese grater device. This deep pain radiates out into my chest and back along my shoulders and taut neck muscles and even down my arms. Apart from this I have pain (a secondary pain) from my abdominal muscles, as if I had done ten rounds sparring with Ricky Hatton while he practises his body punching techniques, a consequence of thirty-six hours of vomiting and retching. My joints all hurt from lying in the same position for thirty-six hours. Curled now in the often-used foetal position I have broken out in a drenching sweat and am soaking wet from head to toe and beginning to chill. I know I have to change my wringing wet T-shirt and pants but the malaise won't let me. The malaise that has stopped me from getting up to pee to an extent that my bladder also aches, the malaise that prevents me from even changing channels (by remote control) on the ever constant day-time drivel pouring from the TV, a TV that I don't lift my head to watch at any point in the forty-eight hours curled up in bed but find the sound comforting and a way of knowing what time of day it is. The shivering eventually forces me to slowly drag the soaked shirt off my back and change clothes for the second time this morning. My mind is in a sort of delirium state now. I go for the pee that I have been bursting for and notice that the colour is dark almost black and it reeks. This is a sign that I am dehydrating and I promise myself to sip more water. I am at that critical point where I have to make sure that I do not dehydrate or go into shock (as has happened previously) as that will mean hospitalisation which I like to avoid at all costs. Back in the foetal position the nausea is back with a vengeance following the exertion of peeing. My imagination starts to kick in as I mentally scream "For Gods sake give me a f***ing break". I am screaming at my pancreas, a pancreas that I hold a vivid image of. He looks like a huge short fat slug with a head but no neck - a kind of Jabber the Hut character with a nasty looking face of that animated germ from a recent TV ad for Domestos or some toilet cleaning product. The face has a

ANDREW'S STORY

look, an indignant smirk that says belligerent all over it. It is green or grey or yellowish brown and the body is covered in weeping sores that occasionally erupt like tiny volcano spewing out steam and a snot-like consistency. Slimy fluid that the evil pancreas is completely covered in. This slime appears to be eating him like hydrochloric acid or something (pancreatic enzymes presumably), and it gently smokes. It coughs, wheezes and dribbles from its mouth and seems to have difficulties breathing or moving. Often I imagine this monster to be strung or suspended on taut piano wires attached to the linings of my rib cage etc and when I move or roll over this pancreas of mine rolls around, gets knocked about against my other internal organs bouncing off my lungs, kidneys, spleen and heart gradually coming to rest uncomfortably on my liver. Sometimes it feels as if it's made of very heavy bloated granite and presses against my intestines and bladder.

This pain is ludicrous now, I feel very emotional. I well up but don't cry I am feeling sorry for myself. Why me? What did I do to deserve this? It's at these times that my mortality crosses my mind, I don't ever feel suicidal at all but I have often felt that death would be a great relief at the peak of an attack. This makes me wonder if you take all your "baggage" with you to the afterlife, your diseases and chronic pain and constant indigestion. Do they go with you? If so, it crosses my mind that I am going to hell either way!

It's been over forty-eight hours now. The nausea
has gone and I haven't vomited for a few hours.
We are moving into the pain stage, the hundred
variations of pain, and the colours of pain. The
many descriptions of pain - light, heavy, nagging,
niggling, aching, twinges, searing, sharp, dull, hot,
cold, excruciating, blinding but most of all
depressing bloody pain. I suffer from all of these
at times and it takes away any feelings of hope
that I may have for the future - a bleak looking
future that is riddled with more ailments like
diabetes, osteoporosis and of course pancreatic
cancer.

"Cheer up it could be worse" someone said to me
recently, which, unfortunately I find very difficult to
believe. It couldn't possibly get worse, I have very
little left to lose (here comes another list) after all
in three and a half years I have managed to shed
the following; hope, good health, marriage,
business and job, social life, weight, dignity,
humour, confidence and finally (judging by this
tirade) my mind. Happy days!

Tony

ANDREW'S STORY

This book is dedicated to the brilliant doctors who have helped us to manage this horrific disease and to the others, in the hope it will educate them.

And to my family, with thanks for their encouragement. They have suffered long in the writing of this book, and also to Anne, but most of all to Andrew.....

Brenda Prentice

ANDREW'S STORY

Chapter 1

1987 In the Beginning…

The office off the main ward that we had been waiting in for sometime was windowless and stuffy. Eventually the surgeon arrived and relieved our tension. He was young, quite aloof and distant. Maybe that was the only way he could deal with giving parents bad news!

"We've removed 40% of Andrew's pancreas, but I don't want you to think that what is left is in good condition, it isn't. It's in a condition I would expect to see if he had done fifteen years hard drinking. Don't expect him to be an old man. He'll end up a drug addict, they all do!" Then he was gone. Andrew was just seventeen!

He made an 'uneventful' recovery and was home in a week. "I'm going to the college dance tonight." "I don't think you are" I said. "You've had major surgery and you should rest." "I haven't seen my friends for ages and I'm going to the dance, if you won't take me I shall walk to the next village and get a bus!" he argued.

He had always been a tempestuous, argumentative child and even now he was pushing his luck. In today's world I think he would have been diagnosed as having Attention Deficit Hyperactivity Disorder, (ADHD) but it hadn't been thought of then. I had long ago stopped giving valid reasons for asking him to do things, as it only gave him ammunition to argue. Now I say 'because I say so' to the usual question of, 'why'? He couldn't argue with that, although he did try!

Eventually I caved in and agreed to drive him into college and he agreed just to talk to his friends, no dancing. There was no need to say, 'don't drink'. He knew what happened to people who had Pancreatitis and had even a drop of alcohol, they end up in Accident and Emergency in great pain. Then they are admitted into hospital for as long as it takes for the inflamed pancreas to calm down again.

The treatment is, 'nil by mouth' to rest the stomach, injections of pethidine or morphine for the pain and an intravenous drip to keep the patient hydrated. Even his friends knew not to spike his lemonade or coke with vodka. They had tried it for a laugh, but soon found it wasn't so funny when he ended up in hospital.

I had said that I would pick him up at 10pm after the dance, but at 9.30 he phoned to say it was so nice to see his friends again, 'give me a bit longer, please!' I picked him up at 10.30 and he was exhausted! Not surprisingly, the next day he was

ANDREW'S STORY

poorly and I took him to see the GP. In front of the doctor I said to Andrew, "You had better tell the doctor all you have done since you came home from hospital yesterday." Andrew said, "I only went to the dance!" Doctor to Andrew, "We don't want you sitting around thinking you are ill, but you must take it easy for a while." Rest was ordered and this time there was no arguing!

There were to be many hospitalisations. On one occasion I went to the ward to visit Andrew and found half his class there having a small, well meaning riot! Fortunately they soon left the ward and it returned to normal. It broke up the day for the other patients and staff and gave them something to talk about, not to say moan! Andrew was given another shot of pethidine and was asleep in no time.

It had all started in November two years before. In 1986 when, at 4am, Andrew had called me from his bedroom, he was in great pain and I gave him aspirin. A little later he called again for more aspirin. I had never called a doctor in the night. Could I do it now? With great difficulty I waited until 7am and called the doctor. "Bring him into the surgery at 9am." "But he has been in a lot of pain since 4 am," I said. "That's alright I'll put him in a side room."

Andrew lay on the couch in the health centre with his eyes shut and he didn't move. It was striking how still he was. Blood was taken and we were sent home to wait for the result. I phoned later to say he was still in great pain and was told, "You had better take him into the children's ward at Grove Park," our local hospital.

They were very kind in the children's ward and also very puzzled. Eventually they decided to remove his appendix although as they said they were not totally convinced that was the problem. My husband Ron and I were sent home and told to come back at 10pm that night.

Andrew was back in the ward by then and the surgeon said there was nothing wrong with his appendix, but they took it out anyway as it wasn't any use to him. There was a lot of liquid in his gut and they were running tests for Pancreatitis. They hoped very much it wasn't that. They said it was usually an illness of alcoholics; he was too young to have contracted it.

The next day we were told that he had an amylase blood count, what ever that was, of 8000. I asked why he was on a heart monitor machine and was told that the high level of pain he was in could stop his heart beating. The confirmation came; yes it was Pancreatitis, what ever that was. We had

ANDREW'S STORY

never heard of it. We were stunned, was this happening to us?

The next day Ron had to get on with some work. We were both self employed and if you don't work you don't get paid, it's very simple really! We had to keep some semblance of normality. I dropped our two other children at school and went on to the hospital where the doctor told me that the amylase had dropped to 4000. I waited all day for Andrew to wake up but the pethidine was doing its work well. Eventually I collected the children from school and went home.

The amylase count was down to 2000 by my next visit and at last my brain was beginning to work again and I asked what it should be.
"I thought you would never ask," the young houseman said. "Low 100's would be nice, in the 90's even better!" "Oh" I said. I should have been able to say something intelligent, but I couldn't think of a thing.

At the reference library I looked up Pancreatitis and read that it is a disease of alcoholics and old men. How could that be? It is characterised by the stillness of the patient and they should be nursed as for terminally ill! ! It was something of a shock and now I did have some questions for the doctors. They assured me it was an old book and things have changed since it had been written.

Youth was on his side and they had every hope this was a one off attack and that he would make a full recovery.

Gradually he began to improve, but the wound from the appendix kept seeping and took many months to heal. He made it home for Christmas and by February went back to school. After all it was coming up for GCSEs and he had missed a lot of schooling. At the end of the first day back his House Master called me over and said, "We think you should keep him at home until he is fully recovered." Andrew was exhausted with one day at school. Later we tried just mornings for a while and slowly his strength came back.

In the following May, Andrew said, "I have the same pain again," and I took him back to the doctor. "Can't have," said the doctor, "You don't get Pancreatitis twice."

The pain calmed down over the weekend and he went back to school. That year he was admitted into hospital 10 times with Pancreatitis. The treatment was always the same nil by mouth, pethidene for the pain and intravenous drip. Sometimes antibiotics were tried, but nothing seemed to help only the passing of time. ECRPs and MRI scans were done but nothing really seemed to show why this was happening. I was always struck by the stillness this disease seemed to impose on its victims. Later Andrew told me that the pain is so great that you do not even want to blink if you can help it, moving is just too painful.

Early one morning the pain started again and I called the doctor. He asked me to bring him down to the surgery. At the time it didn't occur to me that he could have come to our house. It was only three minutes away from the surgery and if he could dress and open up the surgery why couldn't he come to our home? They did know that Andrew was seriously ill. There was some discussion between the doctor and Andrew as to the amount of aspirin he had taken. I was then told that I would have to take him to Grove Park Hospital as I had allowed him to take too much aspirin. He had an overdose and must be treated for it! I thought Andrew was confused as to how much he had taken and he needed to be in hospital anyway because he had Pancreatitis. At that time in the morning and with a very sick child, you don't stop to discuss it.

I think the local doctors found it difficult to accept that Andrew really did have this very rare and difficult to treat disease. They didn't know what to do with him. He always looked so well, it was easier to imply that he was making it up because he liked the 'buzz' of drugs! Well, the test results were there. The doctors knew that, but doubts were planted in my mind. One of the doctors lived in our village so it was all a bit difficult. I had babysat his children many times and I thought of his wife as a friend of mine.

It wasn't easy to think about changing practices but eventually we decided to and this time we were very fortunate. The doctors in the new practice believed him. We had support in trying to do our best for this very angry and frightened young man. In between attacks he was very well and Andrew had got himself a student job and then a motor bike! I had always said he wouldn't be allowed a motor bike, they are so dangerous, but when he saved up for it, it was difficult to say no. We did live in a rural community with no public transport! His sister had waited until she was seventeen, had driving lessons and then used our car. Why couldn't he do the same? We would often get phone calls to say, "My bike has broken down and will you bring the Toyota Hiace to collect it please, I'm at.....where ever"

One morning I called him for college and his bed was empty and curtains still closed. Where on earth was he? His college clothes were there and his books still on the desk but his bike had gone from the garage. Surely he couldn't have gone out, I was confused! The night before he had said that he didn't feel too well and I wondered if he could be in hospital, so at 7.20am I phoned Ward

ANDREW'S STORY

10, his second home and yes, he was there. He had ridden his motor bike to hospital and he had been admitted! The nurse was keen that we should move his motor bike from outside A&E as soon as possible as it might be wheel clamped! She had put a note on it to say the owner had been admitted to Ward 10 but it would be a good idea to move it as soon as possible. Why didn't he wake me or leave a note or, something? Afterwards he said he didn't want to worry us. I wonder why he thought finding an empty bed wasn't worrying.

The staff found it very difficult to see how, if he was in such pain, he could drive his motor bike and they said so. To add to this the amylase was not raised, and I said, "So you don't think he has Pancreatitis then?" "No we are not saying that. Sometimes the amylase can go up and down very quickly, it can be missed." He had the usual treatment and came home in a few days.

*   *   *

April our eldest child had secured a place at Sheffield University to study Languages. We had hoped that she would take music but having done that all her life she wanted something different now. As a member of the Junior Guildhall School of Music in London, we thought she would automatically go on to the college. Each Saturday she seemed to enjoy getting up early and catching the train to London, but maybe she had had enough for now. Should you give children their choice and respect what they want or insist they do what you think best for them? Difficult, we decided to respect what she wanted so Sheffield and languages it was to be.

Student accommodation was something that we all as a family had to come to terms with. As April was late in applying, there were no places left in the university halls. She packed what she thought she would need, sheets, duvet, and towels, and then we drove her north. From the outside the shared house didn't look too bad. Inside was a different story. We took the mattress from her room out into the garden and gave it a good beating. Then we cleaned up the room. It was on the ground floor and had been a double room, before it was divided. It had a window looking out to the back garden where we could see the grass had not been cut all season judging by the length of it. "We can have barbecues out there", she said, trying to make the best of it. The room was just wide enough for a single bed, a desk and dressing table with some hanging space in an alcove. We won't mention the kitchen!

A feeling of abandonment and desolation filled us as we said goodbye to her that first time. The return journey was long and silent, how could we leave her in that awful place, how would she manage?

Of course, like all the other students, she did manage. She may even have been glad to leave the 'war zone' that had become our home for all I know. Andrew was angry and fought anyone who was near and we were too close to understand this. We just fought back and stood our ground. He was not going to get away with bad behaviour or ruling the roost no matter what! (Why don't children come with an instruction book?)

When April had the flu badly and was housebound, the university doctor was called. He took one look at her living conditions and took her in his car to the university clinic. That was really good of him; he didn't have to do that. We were so far away and grateful for his care of her. Later the Public Health department made the landlord put the two rooms back into one. I wondered what made them decide to do a home inspection.

She was charged a deposit for this room and like so many others before and since, it was never retuned. The landlord said it was to be kept as the house wasn't cleaned to a high standard when she left so the landlord had to employ a professional cleaning company! Pity he didn't do that before she moved in.

*   *   *

With GCSEs behind him A levels were looming fast. Andrew was still in and out of hospital, but with a lot of pain medication he managed to cut down on hospital admissions. In the children's ward he was cared for by a consultant that Andrew knew as he rode horses with the doctor's children. Although taking advice from a pancreas expert in Exeter, his care of Andrew was faultless, as was the general care in the children's ward. The children's ward was in fact, several smaller rooms which were all connected. They were light and airy with large windows and had a homely feeling about them. There were many toys for the younger children and other distractions for older ones. Murals were painted on the walls which added to a sense of colour and space. The building was actually an old American war time hospital, so the feeling of homeliness was quite an achievement.

The kindness and sympathy of the children's ward soon passed and Andrew was now in an adult ward with a newly arrived consultant, Mr. Brook. As a general surgeon he also specialised in pancreatic problems, so we didn't have to go to Exeter for consultations any more. The operation in Exeter didn't really seem to have had much effect. The attacks still kept coming and the pain never ceased. The treatment was correct now rather than sympathetic.

Life was difficult for Andrew and that the sixth form college the teachers wondered if all his problems stemmed from his illness, or was he just a difficult teenager. We wrote to the doctor in Exeter, (before Dr. Brook arrived) to ask if he would explain the nature of Andrew's illness to the college.

Andrew suffers from chronic relapsing Pancreatitis which is a rare condition in one so young and unfortunately is very debilitating. The patient generally feels below par and gets recurrent attacks manifesting itself by severe pain, nausea and vomiting with an inability to do anything. In Andrew's case this has necessitated several admissions to hospital and I was forced to operate on him earlier this year. Unfortunately we have no affective treatment for the disease in Andrew's case apart from attempts to cope with his symptoms when they arise. Whilst I would not be in a position to comment on his abilities at school I have no doubt that his disease will markedly affect his progress, both due to the symptoms themselves and obviously the uncertainty of not knowing when he is likely to get a further major attack and be rushed into hospital.

He is currently still under investigation to see whether there is anything we can do to prevent him getting further problems but he is only too well aware that it is likely his disease will continue to run its course with further exacerbations of pain. In the long run he is likely to lose his pancreatic function, become diabetic and require to take oral medication. Obviously this in itself is a daunting prospect for one so young and will undoubtedly affect his ability to concentrate and work at school. Please phone me if I can be of further help.

But he passed his exams well enough to gain a place at Plymouth to study Geology! Did he really think he could become a mineral prospector, hundreds of miles from the nearest doctor let alone a hospital? Perhaps it was more to do with a certain young lady who had gone to Plymouth the year before! There had been no family discussion as to what career direction Andrew might consider. We were just informed that he had a place at Plymouth and he was going!

The Halls in Plymouth were a palace compared to where we had abandoned April. At least I felt he would be looked after if things went wrong. It was 1990, he was 19, and he was gone!

ANDREW'S STORY

Chapter 2

Plymouth and Beyond

Being self employed you need to be a master of your profession or skill and a jack of all trades as well. After the time when other people would have gone home from work, out would come 'the books'. Although many people think that being self employed means sitting with your feet up on the desk thinking of ways to defraud the tax man, actually it isn't like that at all. The fact is, if you don't work, you don't get paid and if you don't get paid you don't eat. Sometimes you could work and still not get paid! Then the tax man will want to know why your income fluctuated. If it has fluctuated by a large amount and if he is not satisfied he will do an in depth investigation. So you make sure your books are in order, suppliers paid and the hundred and one other things that need to be done, are done!

Ron had been a professional musician since the age of 21. He left grammar school at fifteen and was sent out to work even though he was an only child. No exams or higher education for him. He just got on with life. Having saved up he bought a trumpet and then paid for his music lessons. When his doctor heard about it Ron was told to give it up. "It's bad for your chest!" He had a 'weak' chest, and suffered from asthma. Now of course it would be encouraged. So he sold the trumpet and bought a double bass.

He first took lessons from a musician in the Sidney Lipton band at the Governor House Hotel. In those days any hotel worth its salt had its own band. Later he went to the London School of Music on Saturdays, but only when he could afford to pay for the lessons. As an only child, it was a pity that his parents didn't spot his talent in his early childhood and encourage it. He obviously had a gift for music. It has since shown itself to run in the family with his cousin's daughter attending the Menuhin School and becoming a professional solo violinist. Popular music is, like any other, very skilled and needs the same high degree of discipline and professionalism as 'classical' music.

Every Monday afternoon, musicians looking for work would meet in Archer Street at the back of Piccadilly. It was a kind of unofficial job centre. There they mingled and took bookings for work during the next week and got paid for last week's work. 'Fixers' were there to 'fix' a band for a particular job, perhaps a wedding, dinner, or bar-mitzvah. (A Jewish boy coming of age at thirteen) The system ran on good faith and it worked well. Classical musicians would tend to congregate at one end of the street and dance band musicians

at the other. Some would bring their instruments
with them until they were known by the regulars.
It was a good system that served the industry well
for years. Then the police noticed what was going
on and put a stop to it. Musicians were moved on;
it was a matter of public order!

Ron had worked in all the top hotels and
restaurants in London and then progressed to
what was called a 'session musician'. These
people are the crème del la crème of the industry
whether they were classical or pop musicians.
They worked on recording film music, records, TV
and jingles. It was highly paid for the time and
very stressful. Musicians would be booked on the
phone and told to be at a recording studio at a
certain time and date. The music would be put in
front of them and the orchestra would play it
through. If there were any mistakes, it would be
played again. If there were mistakes a second
time, the whole orchestra would be stopped and
the person who made the offending mistake would
be asked if there was something wrong with their
part! Another mistake and you might not work
again!

After we were married, it was important that
someone was at home to answer the phone. One
missed call could be as much as I could earn in
several days. Much of his employment was for
the American entertainment industry as it was

cheaper to employ musicians here in the UK than in America. But after a decade or two, the Americans were going to Eastern Europe as it was cheaper there and the writing was on the wall. The industry was shrinking and first class musicians that we knew were becoming insurance salesmen and barmen. It was a bitter disappointment for them. Others were able to make a living as teachers.

Perhaps the time had come to bring Ron's other skill to the fore. He had always made and repaired instruments, having had training from a friend who was a teacher at the violin making school in Germany. As we knew most musicians in the business we already had contacts. Ron had already proved himself to fellow bass players with first class repairs to their priceless instruments. On one occasion a leading London orchestra toured America. The venues were very hot and then their instruments were left outside over night in the orchestra lorry. The temperature fell to freezing but the next day they were back in another overheated concert hall. By the time the orchestra returned to London, all eight basses needed to be repaired. The changing temperature having forced the backs and fronts from the ribs (sides) of the instruments or splitting the front or back seams apart.

ANDREW'S STORY

Ron also made new instruments and had a full order book. The repairs kept coming in and the order book got longer. We tried employing people but it never seemed to gel, Ron wasn't comfortable as an employer. We decided to look for a house in the country big enough to live in and use for work. It was thought that this would reduce the repairs and give more time to concentrate on making. We looked all over the south of England but house prices went up as we looked at them. It seemed at this time everyone wanted a second home or to move out of town.

Apart from making instruments, Ron had since the age of nine, made model aeroplanes. He had a lot of time off school with asthma and sat with a book by Arthur Mee, which had the plans and instructions. Later he joined the very prestigious West Essex Club, and between all the members they cleaned up on most of the competitions of that time. They designed their own planes and Ron's 'Small Fry' is still used in control line competitions today! Control line is a form of flying a 'plane on the end of a pair of 70ft steel wires round in circles. The stunts performed while going round in circles attracted marks and the one with the highest marks for the best performance won.

After leaving school Ron was offered a job with Keil Kraft, a firm producing kits to make model aircraft. Its owner was also a member of West

Essex club, but his mother wouldn't let him take the job. "You need a proper job, in the office of the Gas Board where your dad works..."

*   *   *

Andrew was still under the care of our local hospital and the new doctor wrote to Exeter updating progress. Exeter replied;

Thank you for your letter keeping me up to date. Obviously there is at the moment nothing that we can do for him apart from try to manage his pain. There are a group of patients with this form of severe relapsing Pancreatitis who will come to completion Pancreatectomy for pain, despite the fact that they are not yet either diabetic or exocrine deficient. This however is a decision that I am always reluctant to take.

Interestingly I was talking to John the other day from Bournemouth who has collected 32 patients with teenage Pancreatitis over the last 25 years and ¾ of these have followed a chronic relapsing and downhill course. He is presenting with the Pancreatic Society and I look forward to an interesting discussion since I think this is a difficult problem which Andrew amply demonstrates.

Perhaps the biggest operating experience of these sorts of patients is Chris Russell. Talking to him

ANDREW'S STORY

yesterday it is quite apparent that about 10% of his patients who, because of pain finally end up undergoing total Pancreatectomy are not relieved of their symptoms, although they are at the same time rendered diabetic. Clearly it is a difficult problem and hoping things get better would seem to be the best course of action.

Andrew came home from Plymouth for hospital appointments. In Plymouth his health didn't improve and nether did the treatment, it was much the same as at home. Not very sympathetic!

What little information we had on how he was doing, came from that certain young lady! I guess boys aren't always the best communicators. Her family home was a few villages away from where we lived. Andrew had met Jane at Sixth Form College. She told me later, that at the dance he went to after his operation, he had danced every dance. I should have known. He never did listen to me.

Hospital admissions now in Plymouth didn't diminish. It was the same routine nil by mouth and so on but they increased his Creon to help with digestion of his food and steatorrhoea.

The pancreas is a vital gland which lies behind the stomach and close to the liver. It produces enzymes which catalyse the breakdown of food into small molecules which can be absorbed from the intestine into the bloodstream. This is digestion. A faulty pancreas may not produce sufficient enzymes to digest the food and this is most noticeable by the presence of undigested fat in the stool which is consequently pale and difficult to flush away. It is also very smelly! It is called steatorrhoea. Creon is a mixture of enzymes contained in capsules which are taken with food to aid digestion. Andrew's steatorrhoea was better for a while after he started taking more Creon but the pain and sickness were undiminished.

By the end of the first year he was far behind in the course and tried to catch up in the summer break, but in the second year he gave up. It was just too difficult to cope. He wanted to stay in Plymouth while Jane finished her studies and he looked for a job. This was at a time of three million unemployed and there was very little choice in the job market let alone a career. As he was not a student any more he had to move out of Halls and Jane shared a house with him. It over looked the estuary and had wonderful views of Plymouth. He found a part time job in an electrical store selling fridges, TVs and so on. He quite enjoyed it and found he was good at selling things; he got on with the public and instinctively knew when to leave people to ponder rather than try to be pushy.

ANDREW'S STORY

Jane got her degree but no job. Andrew was offered a full time job at the Exeter branch and so they moved there. Eventually Jane got a job in a pet shop which she came to like very much. I guess education is never wasted, but..... at least she was working. They rented a small two bedroom house at Exmouth; so they could have a bedroom each! Well that's what they said. I don't know if her parents believed them or not, I thought it best not to ask.

We used to take the children to the beach at Exmouth when they were young. Their favourite game was sliding down the sea wall on to the sand. Generations must have done that judging by the shine on the wall in certain areas. It's a nice little town of many different characters; one part is very old and still has a small fishing fleet. It also has a typically Victorian sea front. There are inevitably modern additions as with most towns, but it still has a railway station; with trains! Eat your heart out Mr. Beeching!

As the name suggests Exmouth is the mouth of the river Exe which rises high on Exmoor above Exford. It collects water from many tributaries as it runs down past Winsford towards Dulverton where the Barle joins it lower down stream. By the time it gets to Exeter it is a large river, at least by UK standards. It's big enough to have had important shipping in the past and still has some shipping today. It is documented that several ships from Topsham, just down from Exeter, were captured by the Barbary corsairs who took the crews into slavery. Over a million white Christian slaves were taken from ships or coastal villages of Europe to build the imperial palaces of North African Islamic states. Spanish slaves were prized above others and singled out for especially barbaric treatment because the Catholics ousted Muslims from southern Spain. The story of Thomas Pellow from Penryn who, as an 11 year old cabin boy in 1716 was captured on his first voyage is heart- rending. He eventually escaped after 21 years of capture and returned home to his ageing parents who didn't recognise him. I often wonder if Penryn has a memorial to him, it should have. (*See* White Gold by Giles Milton).

Today the main traffic on the river is recreational sailing and to sit and watch the little boats racing up and down the river is a good way to spend spare time, I wish I had more of that!

*   *   *

Andrew won 'best salesman' awards all the time. Salesman of the week, of the month and so on. Usually it was bottles of alcohol and they were prized but not drunk, except by visitors sometimes on special occasions! Then he won 'regional salesman of the year'. There was a posh dinner

ANDREW'S STORY

and the award presented to him. He was so pleased with himself. What his bosses didn't know was that his manager let him put down stays in hospital, as holidays or days off for working over time. Without that kindness, I'm not sure the job would have lasted so long. Others didn't!

He was offered an assistant manager's job in Taunton and another move was on the cards. I suggested that as they were both working now they could consider buying their own starter home instead of renting. They thought this was a good idea and began looking at the housing market. We gave them a small sum to help with the deposit and in 1994 they settled on a small two bedroom house near Taunton.

Soon Jane found a better job in the laboratory of a local firm as a development chemist. She was sad to leave the pet shop but she had to move on. While out shopping one day she saw and fell in love with a wedding dress. It was decided they would get married. They had been together since they were both seventeen. I did try to tell her that Andrew would never be any better than he was now. Without making it sound as though I didn't want her to marry him, I couldn't say very much and it wasn't received well. But it had to be made clear that he was ill and he would never get better. There was no cure.

Chapter 3

We moved to Somerset 1972

My parents had retired and wanted to relocate, so when we decided to move they asked if we would mind if they came too. Of course it would be great to have them near and we started to house hunt.

We looked at houses all over southern England. It was a time when property prices went up as you looked at them and 'gazumping' was the order of the day. The house we eventually managed to buy in 1972 was derelict and had a demolition order on it! As this house was an old water mill, it would be big enough to live in and work in once it was restored.

The stream leaked out of its bed and came in through a hole in the side wall of the house and out where the French doors are now! The demolition order would be lifted only if the restorations met with the approval of the local planning office. This meant complying with current planning regulations. Ceiling heights had to be raised on both floors of the house, so the roof had to be raised. The traditional way of building a corn mill is to have three floors and we lost the third floor on the mill end.

ANDREW'S STORY

We know now that we could have challenged the
regulations, but that knowledge came to us too
late. When houses in the village were evaluated,
all the houses around us were rated as Grade
Two listed buildings and ours was left un-graded.
At least we saved the building from demolition and
it's a nice family home inside sixteenth century
walls. Clearly it isn't the same building mentioned
on this site in the Doomsday book. The
restoration would be done differently if we were
starting again, but it's too late now!

Eventually, when we moved in, the repairs had
cost us as much as we had sold our four bedroomed detached house in London for. Looking
back at the photographs, I don't think we would
have that courage again. They say you only do
this once and I think that is true, for us at any rate.

Builders were very busy at that time and had more
work than they could deal with. We were not there
to keep an eye on them and progress was very
slow. Each time we went down to visit there
seemed to be very little progress made. At last I
visited with the children and went home to tell Ron
that we could move in. I thought he would be
pleased with the progress on the house. The
bathroom fittings were in and even if other jobs
were not finished we could camp out in the house.
So we set a day to move and the builders said,
"Do you mean you are moving in?" and we said,

"Yes!" What the builders had failed to tell me was that although the bathroom fittings were there, they were not connected up to water. They didn't work!

My parents had found a house suitable for them in a small town six miles away. I think they were very happy there and joined in with local life. My father took to having a midday drink at the local with all the 'old boys'. The children enjoyed being close to their grandparents who would often 'baby-sit' for us.

I spent many hours in the garden of our new home. It was third of an acre and I consider that big for me to cope with. Well everything is relative and I don't know how people manage with a couple of acres or more! Now that the leat was back where it should be and repairs to the bed of the stream carried out, the children loved to play in it. The shallow water kept them happy for hours. The village was very small, more of a hamlet with few other children to play with. There was a church and village hall but no other amenities, there were no buses or shop.

The children were picked up for school by an old black taxi and it took however many children were going to school that day! Later the route to school was re-measured and found to be shorter than had been thought for years, so the taxi was stopped. All children, of infant and primary school age, were to walk two miles to school in the next village. There are no pavements or street lights on country roads. Progress was coming to the country, well not really!

After we moved, Ron was soon in demand for playing the bass in the orchestras of the area. Most of them are ad hoc and put together for a performance of a one-off concert, show or opera. One year we performed the Mass of Life by Fredrick Delius. Ron played bass in the orchestra and I sang in the choir. Ron was very taken with the music of Delius and belonged to the Delius Society. Soon after we were married he was in bed with the flu and very bored. I went to the library and borrowed two books, one of which was Frederick Delius by Sir Thomas Beecham. It started a life-long interest in the composer and his music. Ron is now the West of England Chairman of the Society.

Nine months after The Mass of Life, Stephen was born in 1978 on St. Stephen's day, 26th December. He was two weeks early and missed Christmas day by a few hours. As April and Andrew were adopted, it was an un-expected joy to us all and Frederick was chosen as a second name. For the other two children it was like having a real live doll of their own. Andrew was a small slightly built child and he struggled to carry

Stephen around. My mother had her heart in her mouth convinced he would drop the baby but he never did. I didn't want to stop anything that would bind them altogether as siblings. The large age gap between the children was no problem until Ron and I wanted to go out and Granny and Grandpa couldn't 'sit' for us. I got a baby sitter in and April was not amused. "My friends at school go out babysitting for pocket money and I'm left with a babysitter!" She was very indignant. But I couldn't leave them with Stephen on their own, so to a large extent I stopped going out! It was easier that way.

At twelve years old, April won a music scholarship at school playing the piano and a half size double bass her dad had made for her. She worked very hard at anything she did. Girls largely do it seems. Boys on the whole often don't so I'm told. Andrew was very active as a child. In fact we were told that he was hyper-active when we adopted him at four months old. He loved anything physical and was good at all sports. He was very proud to be chosen for the school athletics team in the summer and rugby team in the winter. Attending to academic work was more of a chore! Stephen just quietly ploughed his way through life without a care in the world it seemed.

I worked hard to keep the garden under control. No one else seemed to notice! Perhaps they

ANDREW'S STORY

would see it was a mess if I didn't work quite so hard and they might give me a hand. Nice thought but it didn't work! It just got more out of hand until I could not bear to look at it any longer and got on with catching up. There seemed little time for anything else!

The plants in the garden were attacked by anything you can think of, green fly, black fly, slugs, snails, caterpillars, and woodlice. They eat their way across seedlings as though they have been cut with a razor blade! There are pigeons that live in the trees above the garden and think the vegetables are exclusively for them and tree rats with bushy tails, some call them squirrels! Beatrix Potter has a lot to answer for! Rabbits come from the orchard at the back of the garden and occasionally the pigs that also live there, break through the fence to visit us as well. Lately there are pheasants that have escaped the shoot and taken up residence, one cock and six hens!

I grow strawberries for birds or so it would seem. I don't mind sharing but I do think they should leave us a few. After all it's me that look after the plants all year round. Birds can dive though the smallest of holes in fruit cages! It's quite amazing and they can get out again! But most of all, I feed ants, little black ones, red ones and flying ones. I've tried my mother's answer, hot water but I think they can swim. I've tried ant powder of every kind I could find, ringing the changes when I could. I've tried liquid for them to take back to their nests to feed their families and they just love it. After thirty years they are thriving and getting nearer the house by the year. The whole garden seems to be one ant nest now! The children have even abandoned sunbathing in the garden. I thought birds were supposed to keep the natural balance but they don't seem to here.

What we do have in the garden is five glorious, beautiful, mature, weeping, silver birch trees. They are the envy of everyone who sees them but at 60ft to 80ft high they are very near the house, so we have them checked every year. One day we will be told they must come down, but for now we just enjoy them.

I am not ambitious for the garden I just grow simple things like potatoes and beans in the hope there will be something left for us! I can walk round other peoples gardens and say, "Oh yes, we had one of those and it died." Time and time again...

ANDREW'S STORY

Chapter 4

Andrew's wedding 1995

In July the wedding day of Andrew and Jane arrived. It was the hottest day of the year so far with blue skies and not a cloud to be seen, a good omen hopefully. It was a traditional wedding service in a typically English village church. It was the last service the vicar was to take there as he was moving the following week to a new parish. He had seen Jane grow up in the village and was pleased to marry them. It was a perfect setting for a perfect day. April declined the offer to be a bridesmaid as she thought she was too old! Stephen, now sixteen was to be an 'Usher' and I think he fancied himself in his hired morning suit. He certainly looked very smart, as did they all.

Stephen had suffered from glandular fever when he was younger which had left him with a mild form of M.E. Fortunately, having a good share of common sense, he was able to manage it well by resting when he needed to and by avoiding alcohol, which he found sapped his energy. Later he was to avoid going to university. He said he would be thought of as strange to say the least, if he said he was going to bed instead off to the pub with other students.

He stayed at home and attended a local college studying his beloved computers. He was given a part-time job in the IT department at the college he was studying at. That would stand him in good stead when it came to looking for a job. Because of his qualifications and experience he was appointed to his first job, which was at a comprehensive school. Although part time, it was a start and he was the only IT person at the school. He oversaw the installation of a new system which was great experience and I know (as does he) that he was highly thought of by the school. With this behind him, two years later he was appointed IT assistant manager at the local sixth form college with five people for him to manage as well as the system. As he was younger than some of the team, it was his strength of character and personality that brought the team together and he was able to supervise them with little difficulty. The team gelled and was to stay together for a long time. He said, "As assistant manager, I get to do the 'techie' bits and my boss does the paper work, just the way I like it!"

One day he told us that he had overheard a teacher saying, "The computers hardly ever go down, I don't know why we need such a large IT team." The point being of course that the team always tried to be one step ahead of the system so that it never did let them down!

ANDREW'S STORY

We had invited Jane's parents to dinner one night to see if we could help with wedding arrangements. They had things under control and we made a financial contribution towards the day. I was asked to do the floral decorations in the church and the rooms to be used for the reception. We met up again over coffee at their house to discuss the detail of what they wanted. It was the only time we were invited to their home.

Ron had a friend with several classic cars and he supplied the wedding car for the day. It was an Austin 8 and quite a talking point. The children in particular were captivated by it. Many had never seen an old car like that before. It was beautifully polished and had lots of ribbons and flowers decorating it, as they do for weddings!

The reception took place at Hestercombe House, a local country house with a garden designed by Gertrude Jekyll. It had been restored to the original design and the roses in particular were wonderful. The formal garden is in terraces with crazy pavement and plants scrambling up columns. There are little waterfalls and streams with water lilies and gold fish. The Ha Ha kept the cattle in their field beyond the garden with no visual barrier. To the left of the formal garden is a wooded area and to the back there has been discovered a 'lost garden'. It had been overgrown for generations and now restoration work continues to restore it to its full splendour. There are two huge lakes fed by a waterfall some 70ft high with delightful woodland walks and interesting little buildings. The thatched witches' house is made from distorted tree trunks and there are other interesting buildings like the Temple Arbour. Work will continue on it for some time to come.

No one wanted to go in to the reception as it was so nice in the garden. The happy couple looked radiant and I had not seen Andrew look so well in a long time. He always did have a highly coloured complexion and people often would say to me, "I thought he was supposed to be ill!" The Caribbean was chosen for the honeymoon, as it was cheaper than Switzerland, their first choice, and Jane's brother drove them to the airport. They came back tanned and happy. They were proud of their little home and settled down, all was right with the world!

*   *   *

When April came to the end of university, she too couldn't get a job. Even the 'milk round' didn't happen that year and many of the language students went abroad to perfect their languages after their studies. So with no job and little prospect of one, April decided to TEFL in Spain.

ANDREW'S STORY

She got on a plane at Heathrow and left to Teach English as a Foreign Language. She had heard from so many other students how there was a shortage of people TEFL-ing in Spain. She was bound to find work.

She had a room in a hostel to start with and found friends, as students seem to the world over. By advertising in various ways she soon had a few private students and some part time work in Language Schools. It was very low pay and sometimes, not paid at all!

Wanting to move out of the hostel she answered an advert for a room to let. It was one room. She decided to take it and paid the rent in advance, but the landlord didn't move out! She protested that he either moved out or she wanted her money back. After a tremendous psychological fight and with her friends backing her up, the landlord eventually moved out. But she didn't feel safe there and soon moved on. Neighbours told her that he often did this to foreign students.

The economic down turn had also hit Spain and eventually when she came home, as hard up as when she had gone.
At home she took a Certificate of Education, PGCE and a year later started a teaching job in Guildford, Surrey.

*   *   *

Soon after the wedding, the firm that Andrew worked for went into liquidation. It was a national company and 135 shops were closed down. So many lost their jobs but Andrew was employed at once by an electrical shop almost next door. The atmosphere was not the same as the friendly shop he had left behind and when he was offered a job a few months later with a new chain of computer stores, he was pleased to take it.

His health had not improved and he was always in pain. He had learnt how to cover it up, he always looked so well. He used 'over the counter' pain killers as well as those he was prescribed as they didn't control the pain. The doctors and Jane didn't like that and he tried to cover that up too. There were days when I don't know how he stood upright, let alone do a days work. I asked Mr. Brook if it would help matters if Andrew had a transplant and was told it wasn't possible. Then I asked if it would help if the pancreas was removed, would it stop the pain? He said he had never done that operation and hoped he never would have to.

On one occasion Andrew was in hospital and the pain clinic doctor was sent for to 'write up' the prescription for pain drugs. When I visited on the second day the doctor hadn't been and Andrew was still without pain cover even though this is what he was in hospital for. I asked what was happening and was told the doctor had been sent for. Day three and still no pain cover for Andrew. I walked round to the pain department and was told, of the two doctors in the clinic, one was on holiday and that the other would get to the ward as soon as possible but he was very busy. Next day, still no pain cover and again I went to the pain clinic, this time to be told by a nurse that there are other people to be seen as well as your son, he isn't the only one! Five day's later and still no pain medication, Jane told me that she had 'freaked out' in the middle of the ward and said she wasn't moving until Andrew's pain had been treated. A doctor was called from the next ward, a prescription signed and pain drugs at last administered. How could the staff let him do 'cold turkey' in hospital where they should be looking after him? Did they think he was just a drug addict? If he was, it was through no fault of his own and he had many other problems to deal with as well as the pain.

Several months later Andrew was sent to the Plymouth store as an assistant manager. He rode his motor bike to the station at Tiverton and caught the 7am train, returning home at 8.30pm. Two years after the chain of shops was set up, this firm also went into liquidation. This time he was out of work for some while. Fortunately

Jane's job had worked out well and she was gaining promotion.

Eventually, Andrew was taken on at a high street bank. Unfortunately the vacancy was in a town twenty five miles away. We kept hearing that he was to be transferred to a branch nearer home but it didn't happen. It was a twenty minute bike ride to the bus station and the bus left at 7am. It went round all the little villages before getting him to work at 8.45. If it was raining hard Jane would take him to the bus station.

During this time Andrew became diabetic. It meant that the deterioration of his pancreas was continuing unabated. We guessed as much from the amount of pain he was in and the medication he was taking. I don't think the stress of the last couple of years had helped at all. We hadn't noticed the move from an acute condition, to a chronic condition as we only saw Andrew and Jane occasionally. The pancreas releases enzymes in response to the presence of food in the intestine. If there is a blockage in the pancreatic ducts which prevents the enzymes passing into the intestine, they become activated in the pancreas and therefore start to digest pancreatic tissue. This is excruciatingly painful.

When Andrew explained this to me I was astonished. I hadn't understood what was going on inside his body and no one had told me what exactly was happening. I just thought it was inflamed, I didn't understand that it was digesting itself. No wonder it hurt!

Jane began to wonder if Andrew should try to trace his birth family to see if any one else had health problems. His birth mum came from Australia and through social services they found she was still in Sidney. It was suggested that Andrew write to her and social services would see the letter was delivered in a sensitive and sympathetic manner. Between them, he and Jane wrote about his life, marriage and the illness and asked if it was 'in the family'. Through social services the answer came back that she didn't want to know. She might write one day, but not now. Andrew tried very hard to cover up his devastation. It was like a second rejection and all the love and support we could give didn't make up for the hurt. I don't think he ever got over it.

There are groups of cells distributed through the pancreas called the Islets of Langerhans. These islets produce the hormones insulin and glucagon which are essential in the control of blood sugar. As the pancreas deteriorates and the islets are destroyed, the production of these hormones ceases and the sufferer may become an insulin-dependent diabetic. The disease had started at one end of Andrew's pancreas and as it affected more and more of the gland his ability to produce insulin and glucagon was lost.

Andrew was seen at the diabetic department and immediately put on insulin injections. He and Jane soon had a good grasp of diabetes and how to manage it. He got all the gear for testing blood glucose levels (BG) and a 'pen' for injecting the insulin. They had an appointment with a dietician and were told how important it was to eat at the right time in order to 'mop up' the insulin. They also had to learn what diabetics should and should not eat. It was a life-changing regime! He had quite a lot of time off work and the bank was beginning to ask questions. Andrew soldiered on and did his best. He wasn't work shy.

Unstable blood glucose levels put him in hospital many times. A low blood count (or hypo) will bring on an adrenalin rush, sweating, head aches, pounding heart and shaking. Co-ordination can be lost and it's possible to slip into a coma. Sugar must be got into the body fast to bring the level back up. One way to do this is to rub honey onto the gums or give any sweet sugary drink. A high count, (or hyper) will bring on a similar reaction but also with a horrible metallic taste in the mouth and vomiting. This can lead to ketoacidosis (serious blood poisoning which then brings on multi organ failure) which is very serious and must be treated at once in hospital. Extra insulin must be taken to bring the level down again, but not too much in case it brings on a hypo 'low'. It is a balancing act. No wonder Diabetes UK call their magazine 'Balance'. With mal-absorption, sickness and steatorrhoea, it was almost impossible to keep a balance.

Diabetes is a degenerative disease which must be managed properly. Even so, there can be deterioration and retinopathy can occur. With diabetes, digestive problems and the pain, things were not looking good for Andrew. After another hospitalisation, he was put on methadone to deal with pain. It is highly addictive and used to wean drug addicts off their illegal drugs. Andrew said it was like drinking liquidized slugs.

I spoke to Mr. Brook again asking if a pancreas transplant could be considered and I was told that it was very new technology. It was thought a transplant wouldn't last very long and rejection would be a problem, so Andrew would be no better off. Sometimes it seemed as though Andrew was paralysed with pain and we would explore any avenue to give him some respite.

The surgeon sent Andrew to Mr. Russell at the Middlesex Hospital in London for a second opinion. As Jane didn't want to take time off work, I was asked if I would go with him. We caught the train to London and as the train was late we took a

taxi to the hospital. The large terminus confused Andrew, or was it all the medication? It was like old times.
I was looking after him again! He didn't like London it was, "Too big, too busy and too dirty," he said.

The Middlesex hospital was an old building. What a shame that such highly respected people have to work in less than ideal conditions. Mr. Russell had a mild, kind approach and spent quite some time with us. He wanted to know at what age Andrew first became ill and about his schooldays what was he good at? He wanted to know about his likes and dislikes, in fact everything. He asked about alcohol and did he disappear behind the cricket changing rooms with the other boys to drink alcohol? Andrew said he never did drink and doesn't now. I explained that we lived in rural isolation and that if Andrew had drunk as a child, I would have known about it. He could go nowhere without transport and I was the transport! I would have smelt alcohol on his breath if he had been drinking.

The recommendation was that Andrew should have what was left of his pancreas removed in the hope it would stop the pain. As it no longer secreted insulin or enzymes and only created pain, there was no point in keeping it. The operation could be done at the Middlesex or at

ANDREW'S STORY

Grove Park, it was something to go home and think about. We took the underground train back to Paddington very subdued.

Thank you for your letter about this gentleman. He came to see me with his mother. I was impressed by the fact that his first attack was at the age of 15 years. On pressing his mother closely, there was no history of excess alcohol at that stage. Indeed, where he lived made alcoholism practically impossible. Further, I have not come across 15 year olds with alcoholic Pancreatitis. Having said that, anything is possible in this day and age. However, I think the more likely problem is that of childhood or early onset Pancreatitis.

His problems now are typical of the chronic Pancreatic. He is taking increasing analgesia, he is not working and is getting severe pain. The cycle of severe pain, inability to work and increasing analgesia is set.

I think he is almost at the stage where rehabilitation is impossible. Nevertheless in a young man of this age I do believe that the disease process should be interrupted. He is now diabetic. There is absolutely no reason why a total Pancreatectomy should alter this side of things.

Therefore, I suggested that the option of a total Pancreatectomy should be considered. I have told them the operation itself would carry a 1% mortality and a 20% morbidity rate. However the long term results would be no better than 50%. The long team result of his present condition is almost certainly 90-100% disorganisation of his life. Thus a 1 in 2 chance of altering this would be a great improvement.

We can discuss this further in Amsterdam.

*   *   *

At home there had been a phone call from one of our clients who had been working in Italy. Much against his wishes, his double bass had been put in the luggage hold, not in the cabin of the aircraft. He was told the bass would be handled with care and there was nothing to worry about. He got to the luggage carousel just in time to see his bass pushed through the flaps and fall off the conveyer! It smashed the neck off. The man was beside himself as he was hoping to sell this instrument to an American who was coming to the UK to see it. The owner was going to put the bass in a taxi and send it down to us for repair as soon and possible. He also wanted a new cover for the instrument. A very bemused taxi driver turned up with the instrument some five hours later.

Soon after Stephen was born it became obvious that a little more finance in the house would be

ANDREW'S STORY

very helpful and I had to find a job of some sort. As I had not gone out to work for so many years, I had no experience and didn't think I would find anyone to employ me. What did I have to offer an employer? Who could I ask for a reference? I had trained in the fashion industry so we thought it might be good to offer clients a choice of soft covers, made to measure if necessary, for their instruments. I bought an industrial sawing machine and set to work finding suppliers and making patterns. Covers for basses are big and bulky to make. They often drew blood one way or another on a pin or on the machine! But it was a job that I could do at home and the money was welcome. At one time I think most bass players in the country had one of my covers and I still see them occasionally if I go to a concert!

*　　　　　*　　　　　*

Back at the bank where Andrew worked, a lady from human resources made an appointment to see him. She wanted to know why he was taking so much time off and he explained that his health had deteriorated and that he was now diabetic. He also told her about the advice from the Middlesex. She convinced him to give up his job and concentrate on having the operation and getting his health back. After the operation, when he was better and could work again, they would employ him in a branch near his home. Andrew gave up his job.

Jane was keen that the operation should take place as soon as possible. They were seen by Mr. Brook and arrangements put in hand. By now Andrew was quite poorly although he covered it up anyway he could and never complained. Later he told me that he built up a mental wall around himself to hide behind and no one could get to him. The operation was thought to be his only way forward but he was not sure. He didn't really want it. He was just plain frightened of what was happening to him, afraid of the operation, of his future, in fact, everything. He and Jane made an application for Disability Living Allowance, but it was turned down. His contribution to the household budget was incapacity benefit, which isn't very much. With a partner in full-time work there was nothing else he could apply for.

He slept a lot, often fourteen hours a day or more, with the amount of medication he was taking it was little wonder! If he wasn't awake he couldn't feel the pain. Jane would go to work and find him still in bed when she got home. She thought he was being lazy and gave him a hard time. He should at least be up and doing something around the house. As it was she said, she went out to work and then did everything in the house when she came home and she wasn't happy. He had

ANDREW'S STORY

enjoyed cooking and messing about in the kitchen as a child, but she preferred to do the cooking herself so he wasn't allowed to cook. He was left with the washing up which he never liked! What we didn't know was that he was sleeping through hospital appointments and he was picking up black marks! There was no one at home to wake him and see he attended the hospital. He seemed to forget everything but he was good at excuses and covering up. Now I think he got so much 'flak' at home that he didn't say anything to anyone in order to try to keep out of trouble. It didn't work. Jane was grumbling about everything especially the smell from the steatorrhoea as they only had one toilet. I guess the stress was beginning to show on her too. She told Andrew that if he didn't have the operation their marriage would be over.

Jane's parents wanted to pay for the operation privately. It would have been an incredible amount of money but Andrew said no, he would wait. Eventually the date came just when we were going to America for a meeting of the Delius Society of America. We said we would put off the trip but Andrew wouldn't hear of it, "I'll be in hospital for three weeks, time enough for you to go and come back," he said. So two days after his operation, when he was out of the intensive care, we flew to Jacksonville in Florida.

Twenty five members of the Delius Society made the trip from the UK to the US and we were made very welcome. We had a great time for four days. The Campus of the Jacksonville University, where the meeting took place, is huge. The grounds are enormous and beautiful with amazing exotic trees and plants. Also sited there is the wooden cabin in which Delius had lived when he was managing his father's orange grove. It had been dismantled and rebuilt on the University estate. We had an outing to Solana Grove where the cabin was originally built. It was here that Delius heard the plantation workers singing and where he captured many of their themes in his 'Florida Suite'. Delius spent most of his time there writing, playing music and neglecting the orange grove. When his brother tuned up on his way home from the Antipodes, he took over the running of the business leaving Fred free to pursue music.

Fred's father was a German wool merchant who had settled in Bradford where Fred was born. The venture into growing oranges was to keep young Fred away from music. But it didn't work, much to his fathers disapproval, Fred went to the Leipzig Conservatory of Music, leaving his brother in charge of Solana Grove. Father was furious. He wanted Fritz, as he was known in the family, to join the family business.

ANDREW'S STORY

Although I don't much care for the lifestyle of the great man, I do enjoy most of his music. The song, Twilight Fancies being one of my favourites. English music is very special and composers of around that period especially please my ear. You can hear Beethoven, Brahms, Mozart and so on all over the world, but English music, especially in an English cathedral setting, cannot be equalled. The Three Choir's Festival, a great national treasure, has been around since the early years of the 1700's! The earliest record seems to be an announcement in the Gloucester Journal of 12th August 1723. For my money, it's the best place to hear English music!

After Florida, we went to visit my brother in Houston for a week. He had been there for about five years having spent the last thirty years in New England. Now there were only two of us to pay for, we could go to the US a little more often. My brother visited us a lot in England; I think he was a bit homesick really. As he had two children in America, he still made his home there.

We kept in touch with home by email and phone calls and when twelve days later we retuned home, Andrew was out of hospital. His recovery was speedy and he was out just as fast as he could be. He did hate being in hospital, he had been there too often!

Chapter 5

1999 The Revolving Door is Back

For the second time, he made an uneventful recovery! Soon he was taking a little exercise! Jane was in training for the half marathon which she had decided to take part in. Andrew bought a pedal bike and rode behind her when she was out running. They both joined a gym and his strength slowly came back and the pain went. After so many years, it was gone! Someone later described the pain from Pancreatitis to me as being, "Like having a baby every day, without anaesthetic!" This, from a lady who suffered this horrific disease, for many years.

Andrew was still on methadone. It is very addictive and he was now on a very high dose, but he was cutting down very slowly. He didn't tell anyone that he was reducing the dose, just in case he found he couldn't keep it up. Eventually he gave a bottle of methadone back to the GP and announced he was free of methadone. He had done it on his own, without any help. He was still on Insulin and Creon but that was all.

Andrew wrote to the bank to say he was ready to work again, but there was no reply! He went into the local branch and they said they would be in touch, however, nothing happened. How naïve we were to have believed them.

Employment was eventually offered from a medical insurance firm. Andrew fully disclosed what he had been through and that he was better now. They took him on as a trainee medical assessor. After living on only incapacity benefit, trainee pay was welcome. Fortunately he did have insurance and that paid his half of the mortgage. But he did regret not having a similar income to Jane. She was doing well at work and enjoying the responsibility that came with promotion. Now he had to start at the bottom again with a new career. But he was working and he persuaded Jane to lend him some money to buy a new motor bike. Against her better judgement, she did, but was not happy about it. He said he would pay her back. The new bike was his pride and joy, highly polished and never dirty.

The health insurance offices were in a Taunton business park and the new bike came in useful for that journey. It would mean catching two buses otherwise or asking Jane for a lift! The office was new and purpose built in pleasant surroundings but a bit out of the way. About four hundred people worked there. I sensed there was a problem but he said not, so I tried to forget about it.

The brittle unstable diabetes was still a problem. No matter how he tried he couldn't keep it stable and he was in trouble with the diabetes department. They thought he just wasn't trying hard enough. He was always cautious about taking any time off work to attend appointments. He didn't want to lose this job. It was a problem. If he missed an appointment he would be put at the bottom of the list again to be seen in six months' time. Take too much time off work to attend appointments and there were comments! There didn't seem to be much understanding either way! His self-esteem was ebbing away. He put it all out of his mind, stuck his head in the sand and we didn't know anything about it.

And then the pain came back!

He phoned me at 3am and asked me to take him to A & E. He didn't want to wake Jane and ask her, as she had to work in the morning and she needed her sleep. He was admitted into hospital. "What do you mean you are in pain, you can't be, you've had the operation," said the doctor when he did the ward round next day! Did they doubt his word again?

"Where does it hurt?" "In the left side of my tummy and it radiates through to my kidney area in my back." Just the same as ever, had this all been for nothing?

He was sent home in a few days, just as before, with an outpatients appointment and he went back to work. The revolving door was back.

A few weeks later and another night phone call the same thing again. I visited him on the ward the next day and after four hours the pethidine was wearing off, as it would. He rang the buzzer but no one came. Then he asked me to ask the nurse for another injection. I did, but was told, "Ask his named nurse, she is over there." I did and she said, "I'm washing this patient, he'll have to wait, she has cancer you know." Did she have any idea what the pain is like with Pancreatitis? The same analgesia is used to treat it as is used in the treatment of cancer! At least with cancer there can be a curer and people do have sympathy for victims! Pancreatitis just goes on and on.....

I was taken aback. The ward sister had seen me talking to the nurse and wanted to know what it was about. She got Andrew an injection at once and in a few days he was discharged with an out patients appointment and went back to work.

A few weeks later and the same thing happened again. This time, when the surgeon came on a ward round he was with six other grey suited men, all towering over Andrew's bed. I heard him say, ""When did you last have insulin?" "Last night," said a little voice. "How do you expect to keep your diabetes stable?" It didn't occur to me until later that Andrew had been in hospital for nine hours by then and they should have taken better care of a diabetic patient. I had some questions to ask this doctor but he was gone before I knew it. The corridor was empty, I couldn't see him and then he passed behind me. Before I could say anything he said, "You do know that Andrew didn't attend the first appointment for his operation don't you. I had all my staff pacing up and down in the theatre waiting and he didn't turn up. You really do have a problem there!" He didn't stop walking as he spoke and went on up the corridor. I didn't have a chance to ask about the insulin.

What should I do about that? Andrew was asleep when I got back to the ward and I went home. I decided not to tackle him about it for the time being. This time the pain department prescribed pain patches, a slow release patch that should last for three days. The medication is absorbed through the skin so sickness should not affect it. So often the medication had gone down the pan! He was soon out of hospital again, discharged, with an outpatient's appointment, this time for the Gastroenterology Department. "There's nothing more I can do for you," said the surgeon, "Go and see the Gastroenterologist."

ANDREW'S STORY

Home again and back to work. Andrew's whole department was behind with their work assessments and they were informed by management that all employees were to work a long weekend to catch up. It was a bit of a strain but Andrew managed to keep up with everyone. After a few weeks they were informed that everyone in the office was to work a twelve hour a day for a week and then another weekend! He found the twelve hours punishing and afterwards he had to rest by taking a day's holiday which he slept through.

Somehow Andrew never really 'gelled' with the people in the department. He didn't seem to fit. Later it became clear to me that the problem was steatorrhoea. The Gastroenterologist calls the smell 'offensive' and he is right. It has to be experienced to understand and no wonder his colleagues gave him a hard time and a wide berth!

The summer holidays came and Jane and Andrew visited her sister on the Isle of Man where she and her husband owned a shop. There were two children and it was great fun being with the family. They all got on well and Jane and Andrew did a lot of baby-sitting so that her sister and husband could go out together, something they didn't do too often because of a lack of baby sitters. It was a nice interlude for them all and they came home more relaxed than they had been for a long time.

Jane's sister and family had been back to their family home a few months earlier and the children had been christened in the local church where Andrew and Jane were married. Andrew was very proud to be asked to be godfather. He and Jane had often discussed whether they should have children. Would Andrew pass on his illness to any children they had? Medical opinion at Grove Park was that he would not.

But the strain soon showed again and Andrew phoned to ask if we would like to go round to his new place for a coffee! They had split up and he had been moved into a holiday let with just a few personal possessions! Their marriage had lasted just five years.

ANDREW'S STORY

Chapter 6

2000 Devastation

The separation was very disappointing and
Andrew was devastated. Jane had made all the
arrangements with advice from a cousin who was
a solicitor. She drew up the divorce settlement
and took care of the court proceedings. She
calculated the value of their home and subtracted
the mortgage, took away the motor bike loan, the
cost of the carport her father had built for them
and everything she could think of. She also
wanted to stay friends as 'there was no one else'.
She kept the house and all the furniture and
fittings, including the wedding present we gave
them, a camera.

Andrew said that he didn't have the strength to
fight for a fair share. When the cheque arrived
from her it was less than he had calculated. He
was ever the optimist!

I did explain to Jane that it would have been better
to leave Andrew in his home and we would have
bought her out, but she didn't listen. I also said
that as Andrew paid half of all the household
expenses, but didn't earn as much as she did, that
proportionately he was entitled to more than half a
share. That was case law and not my wishful

thinking. Jane was unbending. Soon after, we saw her out with the boyfriend he was much older than her. Andrew said it explained a lot, like the nights out with 'the girls'. She sold the house three years later for three times what they had originally paid for it.

The holiday let that Andrew moved into was at the bottom of a farm track a quarter of a mile long. There was no BT phone connected and his mobile phone had no coverage. If he needed emergency help, he had to walk the quarter of a mile first to get satellite cover and then make the call. If he could use his bike, then he could make it to the hospital without help. The farm building conversion, (you couldn't say barn conversion), was tiny and fully furnished. He therefore had nowhere to put anything, had he received a half share of his home. It was a long way from where we lived and a long way from where he worked. There was a pub in the hamlet where Andrew could buy a meal although he is tee-total. There was also a church and that was about all!

Altogether there were six units and the whole complex was guarded by an Alsatian dog which had been trained very well. It was in no way friendly and kept behind a gate but let everyone know of its presence. It tore my husband's trousers when he inadvertently got too close to the

ANDREW'S STORY

gate! Most of the units seemed to be occupied on a semi-permanent basis, not holiday lets at all.

We persuaded Andrew to get back on the property ladder as soon as possible, prices were rising by the month and soon he wouldn't have enough for a deposit. Each month of paying rent would diminish his deposit money. The only flat we could find for sale near us was a second floor two bedroom flat with a garage. It was agreed that although we didn't want to interfere, it would be better if he were near us in case of emergencies. The flat was bigger than he needed but there was nothing else on the market.

By then he didn't have enough money for the deposit and we made him a loan for the difference. It was a beautiful flat in a new 'village' being built on an old hospital site, a Mrs Thatcher casualty. From the second floor, the flat looked out into a canopy of mature trees and it was like living in their branches, but in comfort! It was very quiet and tranquil overlooking the green. Finances would be very tight but he should be able to manage if he was careful, something he was not good at. His siblings helped him to move his few possessions during Easter and they grumbled that he was leaving it all to them. It took a long time to realise just how sick he was. He usually looked well and he never complained. He simply didn't want us to worry about him so he covered it up as best he could. But up and down the two flights of stairs was too much for him and keeping up with the help they gave him to move in, was not possible. If only he had said, we would have understood, but he didn't. He just went off to buy milk so he could make a cup of tea!

As he had spent all his money on the deposit, he had nothing left to furnish the flat with and took out a bank loan. The first week he was in the flat he lost more time at work and the firm paid him statutory sick pay at the end of the month. It equalled about £42 per week. He couldn't pay the first mortgage payment and so we paid it for him. The next month they didn't pay any government sick pay as they said the wrong sick note had been sent in. His wage slip read £000.00! We paid the mortgage again. Clearly his job was on the line. He really had to try to attend work more regularly; he needed to feel better and soon!

Andrew told me about something called an insulin pump. He and Jane had discovered information about them. I looked on the web and found Input, a charity devoted to publicising insulin pumps. It was started by a man who after thirty years of struggling to manage his uncontrollable diabetes tried a pump and it transformed his life. He wanted every injecting diabetic to know about insulin pumps and to find out if it could be of help to them. The pumps were not available in our

ANDREW'S STORY

area on the NHS. The cost was in the region of £2,500! There was a free month's trial before purchase.

In April, Andrew asked 'Access to Work', a government initiative, if they would fund a pump as it would help him to stay in work. They said they would consider it but the employer would also have to make a contribution of about £300. They would also need a 'note from the NHS detailing his need'. Having discussed it at length with the Access to Work team, it was decided that this would be a test case for this type of equipment as they had not supplied it before. We heard nothing from them and many months later I phoned to be told the form was still in the file and the application had not been progressed! No one seemed to know why. By September Andrew was not in employment and they said they couldn't fund a pump until he had another job! This in spite of their publicity leaflet which said,

'If you are unemployed, self-employed or in a job, Access to Work could help you'.

In December I was told by the Regional Disability Service that Access to Work had made the first funding grant for a pump, but it wasn't to Andrew. We never did get any help from them.

I asked the local MP if he could intervene with 'Access to Work'. He wrote to them but it didn't help. In response to the first information from Access to Work, Andrew had written to the employer to see if they would contribute to a pump, as Access to Work requested. The firm wanted to know more about it and where the information came from and who would provide care and maintenance.

I wrote to the diabetes doctor at the local hospital who answered, '*These pumps are new, innovative and dangerous*' and no, he wouldn't provide the care for a pump! He would not recommend it for Andrew, '*Because of all the complex difficulties with his diabetes*'.

In my naivety I wrote back to him that pumps were not new and they had been on the market for 20 years. He replied saying, '*if Andrew ate properly and injected properly as I tell him he would have no problems!* He went on, '*In any case my department is under-funded and I can't spare the funds to have a nurse trained in subcutaneous infusion care. My department is almost at the bottom of the funding league table in the UK. Anyway, as Andrew had missed his last appointment, it was difficult to maintain any relationship with him and his next appointment would be in six months time.*'

ANDREW'S STORY

I wrote again explaining that there was no need to
have nurses trained as the pump manufacturers
had their own dedicated team of nurses. I
reminded him that as Andrew didn't have a
pancreas and suffered from vomiting and mal-
absorption, he often didn't feel like eating, or if he
did, it often didn't stay down! With a pump he
could eat what was palatable to him when he felt
he could eat it. He wouldn't have to stick to the
diet regime that rules a diabetic's life.

My mistake: this doctor was not going to discuss
things further with me. In a letter to me he made it
plain that he would take this no further and that he
was very unhappy with my interference! No help
there or from Access to Work!

I talked to the man from Input who was aware of
the problem with that particular clinician.

*'There are several people who would like to try the
pump in your area'*, he said, *'But that specialist will
not take on their care. They all have problems
with unstable diabetes, but like so many, they are
told they are not looking after themselves
properly'.*

I then found information in a magazine that said,
1% of diabetics are unstable through no fault of
their own and no matter how hard they try; it is

difficult to manage their symptoms. How interesting!

Input sent a list of doctors who do administer use of the pump and suggested I contacted them. It was also suggested that I write to the PCT and ask for better funding for the diabetes department, so that a pump specialist nurse could be trained. As he said, *'It's not going to happen, but it will bring this to their attention. Any pressure that can be brought to them to increase funding has to be a good thing'.*

A few days' later Andrew's legs had swollen up and I was asked to take him to his doctor's surgery. It was still where he had lived before the separation, some nine miles away. I went into the consulting room with him to meet his doctor as I didn't know him; he was very pleasant and sympathetic and took blood samples which were sent off to the laboratory. But he didn't suggest anything we could do to alleviate matters.

Four days later there was another outpatient's appointment, which I took Andrew to as his legs were still swollen and it was difficult for him to ride the bike. The blood results were on the computer so the hospital doctor was able to view them. After an examination, he announced that Andrew had Ischemic Heart Disease and must be hospitalised at once. There were tears and

ANDREW'S STORY

trauma, he didn't want to be in hospital again; but he was told, *'Well, if you won't be admitted, you must sign a form of non-compliance. If things go wrong, I'm not going to take the blame for it'.*

Eventually he was allowed home to have lunch with us and to get his pyjamas and washing things. He was to be back in the ward at two pm. Devastated; he cried in his dad's arms when we got home I had never seen him so upset before. What else could go wrong for him I wondered?

I thought the best thing to do was write to his firm and tell them what had happened and that he had Ischemic Heart Disease. They had stopped their sick pay long ago and Andrew was being paid basic Government sick pay. He was in hospital for three weeks. Little seemed to happen in that time and eventually he was allowed home with more medication. Some time later his GP phoned the specialist for advice and was told there was no heart disease. *'Tell him to stop taking those tablets. Who said he had heart disease anyway'*? When Andrew's firm wrote to the hospital asking for more information on the heart complaint they also were told that he didn't have it! How stupid it made me look! I know we didn't dream it. We still have the medication boxes. What caused the swelling we still don't know, but it was to happen time and time again.

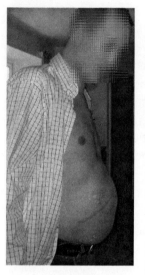

A friend of mind asked how Andrew was doing and I told her that he wasn't doing so well really. I mentioned to her about insulin pumps but said that we couldn't try one as there was no one to look after patients with pumps in this area. She, a diabetic herself, expressed surprise saying she was sure there was someone in her village that had a pump and was looked after at the local hospital. I found this hard to believe and asked her to make enquiries as to who looked after her.

I wrote to the clinician again asking if he knew this patient and who was looking after her. There seemed to be no other way to contact him other than by keeping on writing. I would like to have discussed it with him but he was too busy. Later my friend confirmed that this lady was cared for at the local hospital, where she was employed! No wonder the clinician was angry with me. He had been caught out.

I contacted the acting Chief Executive to ask for better funding for the diabetes department. She had a nursing background and was also a mother.

ANDREW'S STORY

She asked us to meet her so that she could discuss our problems. It was a bad steatorrhoea day for Andrew and during our meeting he had to go to the toilet three times and for once in his life, he actually looked awful. I found her caring, sensible, down to earth and no, I don't think she was made a permanent Chief Executive. Sometime later she died prematurely, a great loss to everyone.

The Primary Care Trust were looking at the funding issue. They also must have contacted the acting Chief Executive. Suddenly out of the blue, we received an apology from the consultant. We hadn't asked for it and I didn't know why we suddenly got it. He assured us that he did his best for all his patients with the highest degree of professionalism. All I did was to ask for better funding for the diabetes department and if Andrew could try a pump! But the apology had a sting in the tail. Andrew was never admitted to the diabetes ward again. If he needed diabetic care it was administered in the clinical assessment ward!

Andrew was back at work, but in early August he fell off his motor bike and was in hospital for a week. He had damaged his knee and later had two operations on it. A lady in the flat below Andrew saw the accident. In her car she identified the silhouette of Andrew in her mirror on his bike behind her. She told me that she was doing about

40 miles an hour and that she expected Andrew to over take her, but he didn't, so he wasn't speeding. When she looked in her mirror again, he had fallen off and was on the road under the bike. Hearing the noise a man working in his garden came to see what was happening. He and the neighbour from downstairs called the emergency service. Andrew's mobile phone was out of range and he couldn't call us. We wondered why he hadn't arrived for tea at my sister-in-law's house and didn't respond to our calls. The hospital eventually contacted us to say what had happened.

"There was oil on the road,' Andrew said, but although we looked we couldn't find any. There was a lot of damage to the bike which was his pride and joy and it was three hours out of insurance! He thought the insurance ran out at twelve midnight but when we looked at the policy, it ran out at twelve noon that very day! He hadn't got round to renewing the insurance. He didn't have the money and wouldn't say, afraid of having to borrow more money from us. Fortunately no one else was involved in the accident and Andrew had to admit that he might have had a diabetic blackout. To actually admit that was very difficult for him.

Several months later he was in hospital for another operation on his knee and this coincided

ANDREW'S STORY

with a dinner we had been invited to by our neighbours. It was their 50th wedding anniversary and he didn't want to miss it! After much pleading he was let out of hospital as long as we brought him back before 10pm; the staff change over time on the ward! Someone had a heart of gold and it did him good to be out for a while, instead of thinking about us enjoying ourselves while he was stuck in hospital, again!

We arranged for the garage to collect the bike from where it was left on the road side. They knew Andrew as he had bought the shiny new machine from them and this wasn't the first time they had collected a motor bike of his abandoned at the kerbside. There was more expense that he couldn't afford, so we offered a further loan and he had more time off work. He was spiralling down fast, his bank account was overdrawn and frozen, and his firm dismissed him two weeks before the end of the second year of his employment. He had no money, was in debt and didn't know what to do.

He filled in a form for incapacity benefit and took it to 'One', the one stop advice co-ordinator at the Job Centre. They would not accept it as it was the wrong coloured form! I took him back to the doctor for another signature on another coloured form, and then took him back to the Job Centre to give it in and hopefully receive an emergency

Giro. That's what I was told would happen, but the office was closed due to a bomb scare. And it was Friday!

I phoned the Social Services and they offered a food voucher which I had to go and collect from their office nine miles away. They suggested that he applied for Disability Living Allowance and that he should go to the CAB for help to fill it in. DLA was eventually turned down. Andrew was very poorly, raked with pain, sickness, dehydration, unstable diabetes and before long, he was back in hospital again.

I wrote to the Council for advice on the looming housing problem but received no answer, so I sent another copy of the same letter. This time there was a phone call in response and we were told, *'Andrew may be entitled to Council Tax Benefit'!*

I phoned the Council Housing department for advice. Andrew was an owner occupier and therefore as he had an asset he would have to sell the flat. I asked where he would live then. What would happen when his money from the sale of the flat ran out, he would then be homeless. What help was there? I was told he probably wouldn't be entitled to any help as, if he sold his flat he would have made himself homeless. He might not be entitled to housing benefit, it all depends. Even though there was a real possibility that the flat would be repossessed by the mortgage company and he would be homeless, there wasn't really any tangible advice, it was all too vague. I asked if he could put his name on the housing register, the answer was, 'he can if he likes but he may never be housed, there are a lot of people waiting. Single young men don't attract many housing points'.

We thought it would not be long before the mortgage company would start proceedings to repossess the flat and it would be better to sell before that happened. We couldn't go on paying the mortgage, we ourselves were now retired and living on a small income. When our savings ran out we intended to sell our rather large house and live off the proceeds.

I called at the Council office to deliver a letter on village business as I was the Chairman of our Village Meeting. A Village Meeting is a bit like a Parish Council, except everyone in the village can attend meetings and discuss matters! With a Parish Council, anyone can attend a meeting but cannot speak unless there is a prior arrangement with the Chairman. There is a time limit on how long they can speak for, usually of two minutes. With a Village Meeting there is no committee, the Chairman is the only official and has to do everything. Should the Chairman ask for help from the residents to assist with some of the work, they mainly look at their shoes! But they do like to attend meeting and have their say!

Two years before, I had been persuaded to put my name forward for the election of County Councillors. One lady had put her name forward in our constituency but there was no opposition and that isn't democratic I was told. So with my arm twisted I let my name go forward. Everyone said I would not win, as the 'blue vote' is very strong, so nothing to worry about there. I was away when the results came through, I had lost by only 500 votes out of over 4500 cast, what a surprise, I nearly got in!

My interest in local politics had come about through Rights of Way issues. Although we were always told how good the public path network is in Somerset, we were bottom of the league table of paths open and easy to use! In 1985 the Countryside Commission had asked that all public paths be sign-posted where they leave the metalled roadway, marked, and be easy to use. There were extra funds available for the work and fifteen years in which to complete it. This was called Target 2000. The only County to reach the target was the Isle of Wight. An opportunity lost and great disappointment for country lovers.

Back at the Council office, we asked for Andrew's name to be put on the housing register. We were

ANDREW'S STORY

shown into a small interview room where a form
was filled in and then given back to us, we were
told, "When you put your flat on the market, send
us the form." Not having any experience we
assumed this was the way things were done.
Later, someone asked me, why did they give the
form back and not put his name on the list. I had
to say, "I don't know!"

Back to the Council again and I explained that my
son was ill and had lost his job and that life was
difficult for him. "Well you could try to get advice
from Shelter the Housing Advice charity." I didn't
know there was a Shelter office in Taunton. I
phoned them and they said, seek advice from the
Council. They have a housing advice line, come
back if you have any problems. The Council had
no significant advice to give; it was all too vague to
be of use.

I rang Shelter again, they suggested that we ask
the mortgage company for an interest only
mortgage but I couldn't see how that would help
as the payments were so behind now and anyway,
he couldn't afford even to pay interest only. I did
write, but several weeks went by before an answer
came and by then the mortgage was even more in
arrears. I didn't understand at the time that we
could perhaps have asked the council for help with
interest payments in order to stop homelessness
and the Council didn't tell us that. I think I was a

bit slow there and missed what Shelter was telling me. The government was bringing in legislation in order to prevent homelessness. Opportunity lost!

Talking to a friend later, she told me, "My cousin's daughter is living in her own house and the Council pay the interest on her mortgage, her husband left her and she has two children, perhaps the children make the difference." But we could have tried if we had known; there's that learning curve again!

I phoned the Council, again a few weeks later and asked, *'what would happen if I bought the flat from Andrew and then let it to him. Would he be entitled to housing benefit?'*

The answer was, *'It must be a commercial tenancy and the tenant treated the same as other tenants would be. This really sounds as though it might be a contrived tenancy. You wouldn't be buying it for anyone to rent, only your son, so it's not commercial.' 'Contrived, what does that mean?'* What it means is, contrived so that the Council would buy the flat for us! "After all," said the man, "Why should the council pay your mortgage?"

What about other private landlords who have tenants with housing benefit, was the Council

ANDREW'S STORY

buying their property for them? How was that different? No answer.

I asked, "If Andrew put his name on the housing list and if he was homeless would he be treated as vulnerable, he is a very sick person?" "Well, that depends," said yet a different person at the council. "Come back when the flat is sold." Is that shutting the stable door after the horse has bolted, I wondered? "Would he be entitled to housing benefit?" I asked. "That's not our department."
.

It's very frightening when you can see your home is endangered and there seems nothing you can do about it. Andrew stuck his head in the sand not knowing what else to do.

We visited Shelter again and they said that there are cases where parents are their children's landlord. It must be done legally and with the same constraints as any other commercial letting. At last, a straight forward answer which we could understand! He should be entitled to housing benefit!

I wrote to the Council and again received no answer, so I went to see Andrew's local Councillor, someone I knew 'of another political persuasion'. She did her best to understand what was beginning to be a complicated situation and wrote to the housing department on our behalf.

The housing manager's letter that came in answer was far from accurate, and the Councillor, having done what she said she would, we didn't hear from again.

Eventually a man from the Council housing department made an appointment to visit Andrew, to assess his housing need. We found him unsympathetic, unfriendly and unhelpful. After arriving he said he had made a previous visit, but Andrew was out. He had left a letter saying he had called in Andrew's letter box asking him to phone, which he didn't do. I pointed out that the letter box was inside the communal front door which had a security lock on it and couldn't be opened from the outside. The postman had special access. I explained that it was unlikely that Andrew was out, more likely that he was asleep in bed as he was not well and takes a lot of medication.

If I asked a question the answer was, *'I don't understand your question',* or *'I don't understand what you mean'*, his ability not to be able to understand simple questions really shocked me. The interview went from bad to worse. He really was so unhelpful. His advice was not to sell the flat, let it be repossessed as Andrew would be deemed to have made himself homeless otherwise, in which case there would be no help. What about the stress that will be caused to

ANDREW'S STORY

Andrew? Question ignored. What about the
money he had tied up as deposit, it would be lost.
No answer.

Andrew's home was warm, comfortable and as
there were two bedrooms, it exceeded his need. If
he was to be eligible for housing benefit, it would
only pay for what was considered to be his need,
which would be based on a bed sitting room, not a
two bedroomed flat. They were dealing with now
and not what might happen in the future. We
explained that it was the future that was of
concern as there was no way in which Andrew
could stay where he was, he was two floors up
and it was getting difficult for him to manage.
What was the advice for the future? Very little
other than to wait and see!

I went back to Shelter to up-date them. I told them
the name of the man who interviewed Andrew,
they said, 'Oh yes, sometimes people come here
in tears after an interview with him, especially
young mums on their own, he is a bully'.

A letter came from the council giving Andrew
sixteen housing points, six for stress and ten for
medical problems. No other explanation of how or
why points are awarded, so I asked for one.
Eventually I had to ask the housing manager for
the information I wanted, it wasn't forthcoming
from the department. We found that points are

given for many things and up to forty can be awarded for medical reasons.

I asked if a doctor's opinion had been taken and was told, no. I asked how many people with Pancreatitis this advisor had assessed. *'Its how illness affects you that is assessed not the illness itself'!* With 16 points Andrew would never get social housing help. I was told the points needed to be in the hundreds to be re-housed.

Later we were told that the officer had *'issued a housing application form which we had not returned!'* It was said that, *'he would arrange a homeless and housing advice officer to visit'*, if he did, nothing happened. We were also told that actually the officer had called on Andrew twice and each time he was out. I did wonder if they had us muddled up with someone else.

I decided to complain about this man's attitude. We had nothing to lose, but it might help other people another time. Our complaint was looked at by the man's manager who said, although they admitted it was a 'strained' interview, (why?) the assessment was carried out correctly and there was, therefore, nothing wrong. No help for future service users there, just a black mark for us! In answer to another letter I had sent, I was told;

ANDREW'S STORY

'It is not the policy of this Council to seek medical opinion' and,
'If your son does become homeless, I am confident that his medical problems would constitute medical vulnerability as defined by the homelessness legislation. He would then be considered for re-housing under this national legislation rather than the 'local' points scheme and it would be the objective of the Local Authority to provide your son with an offer of accommodation as quickly as possible, although this may be limited by the fact that social housing within the Borough area is in very high demand and in very short supply...'

Ron went with Andrew to look at flats to rent, but flat agencies would not put him on their list of potential applicants as he didn't have a bank account or a job. With no financial reference, no one would help him. He said to the agents, "When my flat is sold I will be able to put down six months rent," but to no avail. I phoned the Council again and told them the position and was told, "Try the small ads in the back of the local paper and the housing associations."

Housing associations, a list of which had been sent to me by the Council, all said the same. *'We cannot take any one we like as tenants, we must take people from the council's housing list'*, later that law was relaxed a little and housing associations were allowed a little more autonomy I believe. We were getting nowhere.

ANDREW'S STORY

Chapter 7

Pumper's!

In September 2000 my husband and I had planned a holiday to Norway in my MG Midget sports car, made in 1972. I had recently seen the car in a local garage and thought it was a nice colour, so I bought it! I could not have afforded one when they were new, or when I was young. As we were now retired I thought it would be fun for just the two of us to potter about in. We had decided to take the Midget and follow in the footsteps of Delius. He had documented this walking holiday in a red diary which is now in the Percy Grainger museum in Australia!

I phoned Social Services and asked if anyone could keep an eye on Andrew, pop in and see him from time to time while we were away. I was told that I would have to arrange it with a care agency and Andrew would have to pay for it! He had been granted Incapacity Benefit but that wasn't enough to keep a roof over his head and he said he didn't want strangers visiting anyway. He assured us he would be alright and if he wasn't he would call the doctor. He said he would feel dreadful if we didn't go and so it was agreed, we went.

The ferry left from Newcastle and we arrived in
Bergen the next morning. The old car didn't let us
down as many friends thought it might. We were
able to trace the route of Delius over many miles
and stayed in many of the towns and villages that
he had stayed in. One day we caught a local bus
to Granvin and walked from there along the old
post road back to our pension in Ulvik. Until 1900,
it was the only road to Ulvik. The old road takes a
route high over the plateau; it is a beautiful walk
sprinkled with small lakes, woodland, open vistas.
I had been a walker all my life and although Ron
did not share my enthusiasm, he does appreciate
that to see the countryside at it's best, the only
way is to walk!

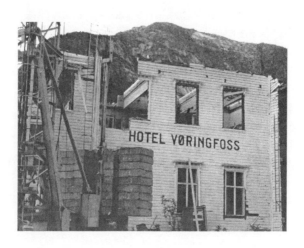

ANDREW'S STORY

At Eidfjord we looked for the Voringfoss Hotel where Delius had wanted to stay, but the hotel had been full and so he went on to Ulvik. We asked at the visitor's centre for directions as we couldn't find it. We were told that if we hurried we might see the last of it as it was being pulled down to make way for a modern building. The young lady who gave this information said the hotel had been built by her Grandfather and she was very sad to see its passing.

Edvard Grieg spent the winter of 1887 in Leipzig. And for the first time, he met Fritz Delius as a twenty five year old student from England. They became great friends and Grieg had a 'nick-name' for Delius, it was the Hardangerviddeman, as Delius had walked across the Hardangervidda. We ended our holiday with a visit to Troldhaugen, Grieg's house on the edge of Lake Nordaasvend, near Bergen. It is quite a visitor attraction and the hut in the garden where he composed, is still there.

Not far from Greig's house is the house of Ole Bull. Born in 1810, he is little known today but at the height of his popularity he toured the world playing Scandinavian music. He commanded a fortune for his concerts and in one night he earned enough to pay for a house to be built on an island that he owned, that's what the story says! The architecture is quite remarkable and encompasses seven different styles. I remembered seeing violin bows in our workshop stamped with the name of Ole Bull, he obviously had a tie up in some way with a bow maker and lent his name to a range of bows, no doubt for a price!

When we got home, Stephen said he had been to see Andrew a few days before and he was OK. We went to see him and he didn't respond to our knocking. We had a key and let ourselves in. He was on the settee, almost paralyzed with pain and couldn't even keep water down. Dehydrated, he hadn't taken his insulin, there was no food in the flat, and he couldn't get out to the shops. He hadn't phoned anyone for help as he didn't want to be a nuisance! He had asked Stephen to bring him some milk when he visited a few days before, but that was all.

We called for an ambulance and the two men who came were so good with him, their care and professionalism was a credit to them and the emergency service. They wanted to know about the pain and I explained as best I could, I also said that sometimes I think his pain is not believed and it is thought that he is just trying it on to get drugs.

He was taken down the two flights of stairs and put on a heart monitor machine in the ambulance, each time Andrew winced with pain the heart

monitor raced. "You can't make that up," they said.
His blood glucose level was off the scale and he was admitted to hospital, this time to the Gastro ward. He soon responded to treatment and a week later he came home, first to us for a few days and then back to his own home. He was lonely and he did miss his wife.

Several weeks later we went to a diabetes day in Swindon. It was run by 'Input' and was for people to gain information about insulin pumps. Here we were able to talk to many pump users known affectionately as Pumpers! Diabetic nurses and representatives of two pump manufacturers were on hand to answer questions and everyone was very helpful and positive. Many people there had experienced poor management of their diabetes and many had also experienced the 'blame game' as I found it's called. When some medics can't cure, it must be the patient doing something wrong.

All the diabetics there using a pump had experienced better management of their condition. In some areas the NHS did fund pumps because it is cheaper to have someone on a pump and their diabetes under control, than for the NHS to pay for frequent hospitalisations. The cost of retinopathy, poor circulation with possible amputation, heart disease, liver diseases, blindness and all the other side effects of diabetes is huge. Later, Andrew's new diabetes doctor was to say, "There is no such thing as mild diabetes."

It was an interesting day and we came home with a lot to think about. This included a question that a diabetes nurse had posed, "Why wasn't Andrew in the diabetic ward on his last admission to hospital'" He was in the gastro ward but he had Ketoacidosis, blood poisoning from lack of insulin. It is a very serious condition not to be ignored... We knew why!

It was clear that Andrew couldn't stay in his flat for much longer. I saw an advert in the paper shop in the next village, one of the alms houses in the village was vacant and a tenant being sought. We talked about it and agreed that I should ask for an application form. I wasn't given the form when I asked for it, the alms houses were only for people who were over sixty and applicants must be in good health! I thought that alms houses were for the poor and needy of the parish but it seemed I was wrong!

The chairman of the alms house committee who had the forms, explained and asked, "Does he have DLA?" "No he was turned down, I guess he is not disabled enough," I said. "Who is your son's social worker?" "He hasn't got one," I said. "If he is as ill as you say, he must have one, I'll find out who it is, he should also be on DLA!" "Oh, how will you find out who his social worker is?" I asked. "I'll ask Social Services at County Hall.'"

He phoned me back and gave me the name of my mother's social worker. I explained there must be a mistake to my knowledge Andrew hadn't got a social worker. The man insisted that Mrs. Wood was both my mother's and my son's social worker and he asked if we had ever had an assessment done. I didn't know what that is, but no, I don't think we have! "I'll ask for one for you," he said.

The social worker knew about Andrew as my mother had often talked about him when Mrs Wood visited her. I think it was Mrs Wood who organised the food voucher for him but I didn't know she was appointed to look after Andrew.

Mrs. Wood phoned me several times to ask questions and eventually the 'Assessment of Young Disabled Person Needs' arrived in the post. It was twenty pages long and covered many things and did reflect his needs, it was very accurate. It said that due to his illness, a stable home environment was needed. I wasn't sure what to do with the report, so I took a copy and sent it to the Housing Manager at the local Council. There was no acknowledgement and I don't know what happened to it. I do wonder if it is still in the file, I'm sure no one ever read it.

It was suggested that Andrew should apply for Income Support, he should ask at the Job Centre!

*   *   *

My father had died at the age of 92 and my mother was living on her own. Life was beginning to be a struggle for her and from time to time she had a week respite care. Having tried several care homes in the area, she thought the one in her village was the best, although none were as good as being in your own home. Eventually she admitted during a weeks' respite that she couldn't manage at home on her own any longer. It was something I had thought for a long time but it had to be her decision, I had tried to support her as best I could but she was fiercely independent and determined 'not to be a burden' on her family.

My brother and I took home what we could of her possessions so that she thought most things were 'still in the family'. My daughter had decided several years before that it was time to 'grow up'. When I enquired what that meant she said she needed a good job and a mortgage! So back to university for the fourth time, to Manchester this time to study for a 'Masters' in computing. For the first time ever, she was offered a job before she had finished the course. After so many starts in life, she could for the first time think about buying

ANDREW'S STORY

a home of her own. Also, she could make use of some of Nana's things. My mother was so pleased that April was able to 're-home' the dining room suite my father, a cabinet maker, had made for their first home in 1936...

Andrew's diabetes remained unstable and he really was struggling with life. He had little money, just incapacity benefit, lowest grade, about £48, it goes up a few pounds after a year, and we made him more loans in order that he could live. Vomiting on most days meant he had to buy a lot more food than he would have done, in order to try to keep the diabetes on an even keel and keep his body weight up. He couldn't make the repayments to the loan company and utility bills were coming in, soon there would be £200 service charge for the flat and he didn't have the money. Eventually he was granted Income Support but it wasn't enough to pay the running costs on his flat.

Desperately I asked anyone I could think of for advice or information. Mrs. Wood suggested that I should ask DIAS, Disability Information and Advocacy Service for advice. I had never heard of them but phoned anyway. DIAS said they would appeal to DLA on Andrew's behalf and that I should phone the DRC, (Disability Rights Commission) about losing his job. I was unsure why I should phone, what could anyone say, he had been dismissed and that was that.

In the meantime I had phoned some of the hospitals and doctors on the list that Input had given me. One was very grumpy and said, "I've got enough to do without taking on patients from outside my area!" Another lady doctor from Bournemouth came highly recommended from Input, but it was a long way to travel! Eventually I spoke to a young doctor in a hospital at Weston super Mare, about 45 minutes away from us. Yes, of course he had heard of insulin pumps and had several patients using them, he would be pleased to meet us if we would like to come up to see him. How refreshing, someone who knew what they were talking about and so enthusiastic! When we met Dr. Knight he told us that he had just come back from a conference in Toulouse which had in part been about managing patients who had been totally pancreatectomised. He later wrote to Andrew's GP that he would be a pleased to accept this challenging patient. He talked about the best way to approach the problem of supplying insulin to a body with no pancreas and thought the square wave bolus might be the best option to try first, whatever that was! Dr. Knight explained what was involved in using a pump and wanted Andrew to have a chat with a psychologist before we went any further.

It was explained that it is important to take at least four readings of patient's blood glucose (BG) level

ANDREW'S STORY

every day, maybe more. Andrew would have to
learn to inject a miniature needle (cannula) into his
stomach area so that it sits just below the skin. It
would have to be renewed every three days. This
is connected by a fine plastic tube to the pump,
which is worn on a belt or in a pocket; it's about
the size of a pager. In it is a file of insulin and a
little insulin is pumped every few minutes into the
body. Some people call it, the artificial pancreas.
It delivers a background dose of insulin night and
day. When food is eaten a calculation is done to
convert the amount of food into units of
carbohydrate, and that is converted into units of
insulin. The amount of insulin is then 'dialled' into
the pump, which delivers extra insulin and the
glucose is then 'mopped up' by the insulin.
Because of this, diabetics can eat what they like,
when they like and sugar does not have to be
avoided. It is quite liberating from the draconian
diet regime of general diabetics. The pump can
be detached for a short time in order to take a
shower. If Pumpers are feeling sick and don't
want to eat, they don't have to. The background
insulin keeps their diabetes on an even keel!

Andrew was not to be put off and we went home
to think things over. The cost of the pump was in
the region of £2500 plus annual running costs of
approximately £800. The cannulas alone were
£15 each and must be changed every three days!
My husband and I would have to foot the bill as

Andrew had little money, but we all thought it would be worth it. Andrew was not happy that we would have to pay but he was convinced that he could take control of his diabetes, so he asked his GP for a referral to the hospital at Weston. Dr. Knight was also a lecturer in medicine at Bristol University and I think was delighted to have Andrew as a patient. I almost felt him rubbing his hands together with glee at the time.

The plans went ahead and the pump was ordered. When it arrived, Andrew went into hospital for three days to learn how to use it with saline. He was sent home for a week to practise and then he was back into hospital to try with insulin. He took to it like a duck to water and his blood glucose stability was improving. Within three days the readings were more stable than they had ever been. Andrew was so pleased, he didn't phone the nurse or doctor as all seemed to be well. They, on the other hand, were concerned that they hadn't heard from him! We went back a week later and adjustments were made but basically all seemed to be well.

A few weeks later I phoned the GP but I was not put through. He was busy and I asked for him to phone me. Nothing happened so I phoned again. After the sixth time of phoning my husband said, "He is not going to phone you." "Why shouldn't he?" I said. "I don't know, but if he was going to phone, he would have done it by now!" "Strange," I thought.

We had told Andrew that we would ask the Primary Care Trust to fund the pump as they do have a committee to consider miscellaneous items, although we didn't expect them to pay for it. We hoped it would make him feel better about the funding of it all. The PCT apparently wrote to the GP for an opinion and he passed the letter on to the diabetic doctor at the local hospital. He wrote to the PCT saying that Andrew's BG was *worse* on the pump than it had been before it was used! We didn't hear from the PCT. We also didn't know that this is what had happened until several years later, when we looked at the hospital notes at Grove Park. As far as we could see, the pump was a great improvement. We also found in the notes a letter in which the GP said he was unhappy about the *'unpleasantness's'* between the doctor at the local hospital and me! That's why he wouldn't speak to me on the phone all that time ago!

I suggested to Andrew that he changed doctors as nine miles was a long way for me to take him when he wanted to go to the surgery. There was a surgery in the next village with a main health centre in town and he could catch a bus there, so he changed. It pleased him to think he could go to the doctor's without having to ask me for a lift every time. Andrew asked me to go with him to the first meeting with the new doctor as he wanted company and support. I felt the doctor seemed a little bemused at the long list of medication Andrew said he was on. I went to collect Andrew to take him to the next appointment but he was very poorly with pain and steatorrhoea. He didn't want to be too far away from a toilet and wanted to cancel the appointment. I thought I had better keep the appointment and tell the doctor how things were. The doctor said, "Andrew makes an appointment and you keep it for him, hmm!" He didn't offer a home visit; in fact, he never did make a home visit and had no advice, he had nothing to say at all. Oh dear!

Several years later this doctor came when Andrew was living with us, it was an 'out of hours' call as Andrew was in great pain. The doctor offered a paracetamol! After he left, I took Andrew to A & E and he was given morphine.

Although Andrew was very upset at the thought of having to move from his home again, it had to be put up for sale. The housing market had risen so he would gain financially out of it, but he would have preferred to keep his home. He didn't know what he would do when it was sold. He couldn't rent and he couldn't support a mortgage. And the Social Worker said he needed a stable environment!

ANDREW'S STORY

Again we asked the Council for advice, *'he can present himself as homeless if he likes but if he sells his home he has made himself homeless'*. We had been here before! With sixteen points he was not going to be housed.

Chapter 8

Another new home.

The Disability Information and Advisory Service
(DIAS) made an application for the DLA appeal.
The lady who dealt with this said that Andrew had
a hidden disability, just as she had. *'Because you
can't see it, it doesn't mean it isn't there. Anyone
who cannot absorb nourishment from food
naturally, without intervention, is severely
disabled'*. Andrew had never thought of himself as
disabled in that way, he had two arms and legs
and wasn't in a wheel chair so didn't think of
himself in that light. In fact, it was hard for him to
admit he was disabled at all. He had been turned
down by DLA so he couldn't be!

I phoned the Disability Rights Commission and
told them that DIAS had suggested that I phone
them. They wanted to know about Andrew's
health and about the way he had lost his job.
They told me that all firms over a certain size
must, by law, employ a percentage of disabled
people. Diabetes is considered disabling in
employment terms, without the other health
problems. They were sure Andrew would have
been considered as disabled. They asked what
adjustments had been made! I didn't know what
they meant and when they explained I said, "None

as far as I know." It was a bit of a shock to Andrew as no one had said anything about being employed as disabled. It wasn't on his employment contract as far as he knew.

The DRC explained that they would like us to take this case to an employment tribunal. They could not do it for us, but would give all the help and advice we would need to do it ourselves. They wanted to give a 'shot over the bow' to this firm to make sure they didn't treat anyone else in this way in the future. Andrew and I talked it over, he said he could not do it himself but asked if I would do it for him. He felt so unwell with pain and all the other problems that on some days he didn't get out of bed. I agreed and said I would do my best to try to understand matters and deal with them for him.

The flat was put on the market and the manager of the Estate Agency turned out to be someone Andrew knew from school. The flat was soon sold to a first time buyer who was in the Army. The sale should have gone through quickly but it took months. The buyer's solicitor really made a meal out of the conveyance. We thought the completion was in sight at last when, she asked us about the preservation orders on the trees on the Green! We didn't know anything about that, what did that have to do with us? We might have been forgiven for thinking she was being paid per letter!

The sale was held up again for weeks. The manager of the Estate Agency was embarrassed and we asked for the flat to be returned to the market. He said he would do that as the buyer's solicitor was prevaricating for what reason he didn't know. However, with that, they exchanged contracts and a date was set for completion. It needed to be over for Andrew's sake, it wasn't doing him any good with this hanging over him. He was depressed enough at losing his home again, without the process being so prolonged.

A couple of weeks later I called to see Andrew on my way out shopping and I wondered if I could get him anything. No answer to my knocking so I let myself in. He was in a dazed state on the floor. I asked, "What on earth are you doing?" And he said, "I'm not sure, I don't think I'm very well." I wasn't very amused and said, "If you aren't well why didn't you call someone?" "I think I did, I think I phoned the 'Out of Hours Service'." "Andrew, don't you know, either you did phone or you didn't!" I was a bit exasperated. Why wouldn't he ever call if he was not well? "I'm sure I did, but they didn't come," he said. I thought he was just making an excuse for not doing anything to help himself and I was annoyed. "'Well, would you like me to phone and see what happened?" And to my amazement he said, "Yes."

ANDREW'S STORY

I phoned the Out of Hours Co-operative Service and asked if there had been a call from Andrew in the night. A doctor took the call, not the receptionist and identified himself; he said he would look up the computer. Rather curtly he said, "Yes at 12.30am. He was phoned back at 2.30 and 4.30 and 8am but he didn't answer so I guessed he was alright." I was shocked and said, "As he didn't answer, didn't it cross your mind there could be something wrong?" "If there was, his wife would have rung back." I asked, "What wife?" Silence for a moment, then, "I thought Andrew was married, does he live on his own then?" "Yes." "Oh, well I've only just come on duty I haven't been here all night, what's wrong with him?" I said quietly and slowly, "I don't know what's wrong with him, I am not a doctor! He's not well and I think I had better take him home with me. He can't be left on his own."

I told Andrew what was said and he asked who the doctor was. When I told him he said, "I'm not surprised by his attitude, he is one of the partners at the Wellington surgery that I've left, I never did get on with him, he doesn't believe I have Pancreatitis, he thinks I'm a junky."

With hindsight it seems that Andrew may have had a nocturnal hypoglycaemic episode, which can be very dangerous, he certainly was ill. I wrote to the Out of Hours Office and made a complaint. It was acknowledged and I waited for an answer…

*   *   *

A small one bedroom ground floor ex-council flat came on to the market and we decided to mortgage our house and buy it for Andrew. We just couldn't see him living on the streets, homeless, in a cardboard box. It wasn't his fault he was in this trouble. There was an overlap between Andrew moving out of his flat and into the new one, so he put his things in storage and came home to us for a few weeks. He tried very hard to fit in and not be a nuisance. There was none of the turbulent teenager left in him. Without us asking, he smoked outside in the garden and respected our wish for a smoke free home. He always had the TV on which drove us mad, so we all had to be tolerant of each other. Andrew's sleeping patterns were all over the place. Sometimes I would find him at two in the morning sitting in the kitchen with the TV on, fast asleep!

Now that he had some money, Andrew had carpets laid in the new flat and moved in. He had to dispose of some of his furniture and the curtains didn't fit. There wasn't room for his dining table and chairs; he thought he could eat off the coffee table by sitting on the floor! Otherwise a tray on his knee would be sufficient, down sizing was

ANDREW'S STORY

difficult and painful! The flat was near that village's surgery; local shops and a bus passed the door, which was a bonus!

He opened a bank account with the proceeds of the sale of his flat and paid off the bank loan for the furniture that he didn't have any more and he paid us. He could now pay the running costs of the pump, which relieved him greatly as he hated us having to pay for it. With financial advice from CAB he paid what he could, there were many debts, but he had to have some money to pay us rent, as without that we couldn't pay our mortgage. At times he was very poorly and even if he was out of bed he could not go out of the flat very far. We began to shop for him sometimes and if he hadn't been to the post office or bank he couldn't pay us. So we kept the till rolls and disposed of them when he paid the bill.

Through all this time the doctor never came to see him. I had to remind Andrew about hospital appointments and see he got there. Now that he had moved again I suggested that he change doctors as the last one wasn't interested in him. On good days Andrew could walk to the Health Centre in this village so he re-registered again. He was now back with the practice we had left so long ago and his new doctor was our neighbour who had known Andrew since he was a child. Perhaps things would improve now?

*　　　　　*　　　　　*

The DRC were very busy and all their solicitors were fully occupied but again they stressed they did want us to challenge the dismissal. They allocated us a private firm of solicitors in Cardiff, Russell Jones and Walker and a young lady, Juliet, prepared the case. Although we never met Juliet, she guided us through the maze of the tribunal appeal with great skill. We spoke frequently on the phone and the process started by Andrew filling in an initial interview form of nine pages, which Juliet sent to us. From this, she set out our application to the Employment Tribunal. The form covered eighteen subjects, most with sub headings, starting with;

* The applicant is a disabled person under Section 1 of the Disability Discrimination Act of 1995!

(Confirmation, he is disabled, why didn't anyone ever tell us? Surely the doctor should have told us)

* The applicant has the physical impairments of diabetes and Pancreatitis

* The applicant has the mental impairment of depression. This is a clinically well-recognised

mental illness and is recognised by a respectable body of opinion.

* The applicant's impairment has more than a minor or trivial adverse impact in that the applicant has to carry out normal activities in a different way to persons without impairment!

And then she listed five difficulties in carrying out day to day activities.

I couldn't believe what I was reading; someone who understands what is going on and can put it in such clear terms. Someone on our side, at last! She then described how the impairments would affect the day to day activities without medication.

* Mobility * Continence * Memory. All with examples.

The facts are that the applicant disclosed details of his medical condition when he applied for the position and were contained in his curriculum vitae.

He was unjustifiably treated as he was dismissed after a written warning.

The respondent is in breach of Section 5 (2) in that it failed to make reasonable adjustments in respect of the following:

- Failing to interview to discuss steps that could assist;
- Failing to adjust employment policies or practise, for example the sickness procedure.
- Failing to transfer to an existing vacancy.
- Failing to reallocate duties to accommodate times when the applicant's condition worsens.
- Failing to provide or contribute to the provision of an insulin pump.
- Failing to adjust working hours or consider part time working.
- Failing to consider working from home by computer.

The applicant seeks the following; a declaration that the Respondent unlawfully discriminated against the Applicant in breach of the Disability Discrimination Act 1995 and compensation.

Well! What a surprise! I didn't understand just what had been involved. No wonder the DRC wanted us to take this further.

Then the Questionnaire of the Person Aggrieved sent to the employer.

The questions included,

ANDREW'S STORY

- Do you accept that my statement is an accurate description of what happened? If not in what respect do you disagree?
- Do you accept that I am a disabled person within Section 1 of the Disability Discrimination Act? If not please state your reasons in full.
- Please confirm that I informed the Company of the material features of my condition at my interview and in my curriculum vitae.
- Please provide full details of any reasonable adjustments that were considered by the Company.
- What steps were taken to obtain government funding or other funding towards the cost of relevant adjustments? If none, why not?
- What training has the Company given to training its staff on disability issues, (the staff members were named).

And so it went on for 4 pages ending with,

NB- by virtue of Section 56 of the Act this questionnaire and any reply are admissible proceedings under the Act.

There were exchanges and phone calls, phone conferences with the Employment Tribunal and these went on for almost a year.

After one phone conference we received a 'case management order' from the Employment Tribunal with a footnote. It said;

Note.

I am seriously concerned at the prospect of the applicant proceeding with this case without legal assistance. Russell Jones and Walker have been helpful within their instructions from the Disability Rights Commission but this is a difficult case to prepare because of the medical implications and some form of legal assistance for the applicant would greatly help both parties and the tribunal. I cannot make any direction but I hope the comment will be of use to the applicant in any application for such assistance.

Within four weeks of this and the date set for the hearing, the Company backed down and settled. The compensation was not great but it was victory for us, for the DRC and for Juliet, without whom I could not have managed. There was a proviso that there would be no publicity. Andrew was disappointed about that, but dealing with this was a struggle for me and I was relieved that it was over. I've often wondered what would have happened had the newspapers got hold of the story.

ANDREW'S STORY

Chapter 9

Just a nuisance or more?

The Out of Hours Co-operative Service responded at last!

'My apologies for the delay in writing to you after our phone call. I am afraid there were a number of factors that prevented me contacting you earlier. I would like to explain what I have learnt in relation to your original complaint, outline those changes that have occurred in the interim with arrangements for handling complaints and other steps taken to improve the quality and systems operated and finally the suggested information to be available to the doctors on duty if Andrew calls again.

The original call from Andrew was triaged by the nurses, the call and information was then passed to the doctor working overnight. I have spoken to the doctor concerned who informs me that the message was that Andrew was in pain from continuing pancreatic problems. There was no expectation that unconsciousness was a risk. The doctor tried to phone back but as there was no answer assumed that he had fallen asleep. With hindsight a different conclusion might have been drawn. A message is now on the computer to aid any duty doctor in the future.

In order to speed up the response and to manage complaints in the most sensitive way any complaints resulting from Out of Hours Co-operative Service will be handled by the patients own practice. The practice manager can approach other agencies involved and explain the circumstances and findings to the patient. This approach will help the patients GP to involve the parties of any problems and correct changes can be made. A member of our committee is already at work reviewing our systems to ensure that our standards are improved wherever possible. This is a new initiative but one that we will continue as part of our desire to maintain and improve the quality of our care.

The following will appear on the computer.

'Andrew has severe chronic Pancreatitis and diabetes. He has an insulin pump inserted. He suffers a lot of pain and is currently taking oxycontin, dihydrocodeine. He takes zopiclone, gabapentin and some over the counter analgesics, he attends the pain clinic. There have been occasions when the pain is more severe than usual and he has requested pethidine injections'.

ANDREW'S STORY

Once again, may I say I am sorry that the original problem occurred and for the delay in my reply, I hope you will agree that there are a number of actions taken that will hopefully prevent this situation arising again.'

We were very satisfied with the response, the chairman couldn't have taken more care or effort and we were happy with that.

The computer advice was a good attempt to get to grips with the medication; they only missed out creon and amitriptyline! As for the over the counter medication, one was nytol which is very addictive and in my opinion should not be on sale without a prescription…

*   *   *

After moving to the small one bedroom flat that we had bought, it was suggested that Andrew apply for housing benefit. The form was filled in and taken to the department and we heard no more. Several weeks later an enquiry revealed that no form was recorded and they said it hadn't been handed in! I suggested that Andrew should ask the Citizens Advice Bureau for help with the housing benefit department.

My two other children are computer 'whiz-kids' and they came up with websites for us all to read, but Andrew was not interested, he found the concentrating difficult. Reading anything more than a light magazine was beyond what he wanted to do. He would concentrate if it was really necessary but otherwise not. It gave him a headache.

I joined the Pancreatitis Supporters Network (PSN). This website is very informative and I leant so much from it. It was set up by a man and his wife to help other people who found themselves in the same position that we were in. At one time they had been in education and social services, which was before Pancreatitis changed their lives.

There is a communication board on the site and I began to read other people's stories, many of which were similar to ours. How often they are treated by professionals with no experience of this disease. And how often they are treated as though they are simply alcoholics or drug addicts trying it on. You couldn't really blame the doctors; it was their training and education that needed to be updated.

Quote from the PSN.

'Firstly, and quite importantly, I don't drink alcohol, I never have, I don't even like the taste. The reason I mention this is because it seems that every leaflet to do with Pancreatitis makes the

ANDREW'S STORY

assumption that your continued suffering is your own fault and is due to alcohol abuse and that Pancreatitis goes away when you stop abusing alcohol. In my experience the same teaching has rubbed off on nurses, many of whom treat me as a second class citizen, to the point where I now avoid treatment.

I believe my condition is related to my genes. My grandfather died from kidney failure when my dad was three months old. His brothers both died before they were 30… from kidney failure. Dad is diabetic and has steatorrhoea and nausea but doesn't seek medical treatment. If he has Pancreatitis it is not severe!

In 2000 while visiting friends I began to feel very ill. I was in a lot of pain, abdominal going through to the back (sound familiar?) and had been violently sick. I don't need to tell anyone how painful being repeatedly sick is when there is nothing to come up and the bile is burning the back of your throat. My distressed partner called the ambulance and after a huge wait I was seen by some kid on work experience… pretending to be a JHO. This doctor told me the most likely cause was….. Constipation! I asked for a second opinion and was told it is the middle of the night, there isn't anyone! Back at the hotel I continued to be repeatedly violently sick. The pain just got worse and in the morning we got a taxi home.

That afternoon my GP had me admitted to hospital and after the usual X-rays, scans, blood test, cameras down throats etc. the diagnosis was made, Pancreatitis. Over that year I was in and out of hospital twelve times and the treatment was just morphine, cyclizine and a drip. I had to be careful that I didn't ask for morphine when I was in pain as assumptions were being made that not only was I an alcoholic but also a heroin addict willing to fake an illness to get free drugs! I signed myself out of hospital a few times when I could barely stand up, just because I was so sick of how I was being treated.

Eventually, the way I was treated changed and I believe a senior doctor made it clear that I didn't drink and as the nurses got to know me they realised that I wasn't after the morphine. I remember once having been in agony for five hours the sister coming to ask me if I wanted morphine, without me having to beg for it! It was only then that I was told I had been written up for 20mg every hour if needed. Diamorphine was also offered if I felt my pain was bad enough. Since then my trips to hospital have been less frequent and I haven't left until I have been discharged and can eat etc. I don't like hospitals no matter how friendly the staff are now and I still have nightmares that I'm having metal cameras shoved down my throat.

ANDREW'S STORY

I have problems getting to sleep at night because of the pain, when I do get to sleep I need at least ten hours or more if have done anything the day before. It's difficult to know what warrants painkillers or a call to the GP or the hospital, or ambulance as my condition can change rapidly.

I don't plan holidays now as I don't want to end up in a strange hospital being made to feel that somehow my illness is all my own fault. It annoys me taking about thirty tablets a day. The last thing you want to attempt is swallowing pills when you wake up feeling very very sick. I'm not sure what is the worst, constant pain or constant nausea!'

Andrew's health was slowly deteriorating. The morphine tablets that he had been put on didn't cover the pain any more, the problem is that the body gets used to it and then needs more for the same effect. The dose was not increased and if it was a bad sickness day, the tablets sometimes ended up down the toilet. He was only given weekly prescriptions. So, short of medicine, he would ask for extra tablets from the GP or if it was night time or weekend when he ran out, he had to phone the out of hours service for pain cover. The service had changed from the local co-operative to a full NHS controlled service. To start with the service was fine but slowly it declined.

It appeared to me that the medics were seeing this simply as a ploy on Andrew's part to obtain more morphine, just like a drug addict. I began to understand what the doctor had meant, so long ago when he said, "He will end up a drug addict, they all do." It was not seen for what it was, someone in great pain trying to get help.

The out of hours system works like this, you phone the NHS Direct and a receptionist takes your details saying a nurse will ring back to assess your need. The nurse will eventually call back and take your details and assess your need. Then, if they think it necessary they say the doctor will phone you back and also assess your need. The doctor will eventually call and take your details. He may say he will visit you at home or invite you to the emergency centre, which is not easy without transport. Occasionally they would come and give a shot of pethidine; other times they may advise you to call the ambulance service. This all takes a very long time, especially when the pain is excruciating and won't go way.

Sometimes Andrew would call the ambulance and end up in Accident and Emergency. The time to treatment would depend on how busy they were and their assessment of the severity of his condition. If he was not kept in, he would phone us for a lift home. This happened once when we were away and at 4am he was discharged from

ANDREW'S STORY

A&E. He had to get a taxi home and it cost £40 at that time in the morning! If only they had let him rest for a few hours he could have caught the bus.

From the PSN

'Newcomer, it's the first time I have posted.

This time last week I was being driven in an ambulance to the local
A&E with a pain from hell, it happened exactly six months ago for the first time. Now I am waiting for investigations to see exactly what's up but I feel sure it's Pancreatitis. I had my gallbladder out seventeen months ago and was told that there was calcification somewhere in the pancreas. What jumped out at me about the messages is the feeling that people were thinking you are a junkie, that is exactly how I have felt both times and it is so upsetting. I and all of us with this wretched thing have far better things to do with our time. I'm a staff nurse and I am self employed through an agency so it's really worrying me about what to do for money when I'm sick. The only pain relief that seems to work for me is morphine when I have a really bad attack. The only people who seem to be sympathetic were the ambulance crew!'

Dr. Peter the GP now began to be very difficult about prescribing for the pain and Andrew was referred back to the pain clinic, there was a long wait for an appointment. When it came, I attended the appointment with him and we went through all the different medications that had been tried. Andrew was told they couldn't give stronger medication and he must try harder to make do with what he had.

One Friday afternoon Andrew asked me to take him to the surgery in the village; the only doctor on duty was a young lady locum. Andrew told her about not having a pancreas, the sickness and that he had no pain cover for the night, I'm not convinced she was familiar with the disease at all. She gave a prescription for medication and we took it to the practice pharmacy next door. The pharmacist said that Andrew was not to have any more pain medication as he had had his week's supply. Andrew was trying it on with the new doctor as she didn't know any better. We were ushered back into the surgery where the new doctor said she couldn't help us; the prescription (which I had signed) was taken away. I asked what Andrew was to do for pain cover over night and she said she didn't know! Come back tomorrow and see the other doctor. Andrew went home and said he would take double sleeping pills and try to sleep through the night so as not to have to go to the Out of Hours Service again! I didn't sleep much that night, but he didn't phone. Saturday morning and we went back to the surgery; a very correct and distant doctor gave enough cover for two days. Come back on Monday!

A few months later Andrew was seen in the pain clinic again and was told he could have short term 'breakthrough' morphine as well as the long term that he was already on. Pity he didn't say that the last time we saw him! We were seen by the pain doctor again a few months later and this time, the pain psychiatrist and an acupuncturist also attended the appointment. Three of them, I was glad to be with Andrew to help him cope with three people quizzing him, they never seemed too sympathetic. It was agreed that Andrew would be seen by the psychiatrist and the acupuncturist. There was no other help to relieve the pain other than what had been prescribed previously. They couldn't keep increasing the medication, it couldn't keep going up and I don't think they believed he was vomiting up the pills on a fairly regular basis.

One night as I sat in the car park of the Out of Hours doctors, Andrew come out in tears. When he got to the car he said he had just been told that he was a waste of NHS resources! I wanted to go back and see the doctor but he asked me not to, "Just take me home please." After that he asked me to go in with him if he had to visit the A&E or out of hours, not just to be the taxi. How awful that he felt he must take his ageing mother with him in order to stave off hurtful unnecessary remarks, often with insinuations that he was just a drug addict trying it on. He had been smoking a little but now he began to smoke more heavily.

I took my concerns to the out of hours service providers and they asked the GP to put some details of Andrew's condition on their computer again, (what happened to the last ones I wondered), to give some guidance to the doctors. This done, things improved for a while and on occasion there would be a doctor on duty who did understand the problems of Pancreatitis. Their kindness and concern would have me almost in tears and I realized that I had been unconsciously waiting for their innuendos. I was so relieved when it didn't happen! I wondered how Andrew felt about it after nearly eighteen years, or perhaps I really knew. Suggestions that Andrew should be hospitalised were usually turned down, he couldn't stand the thought of more drips in veins that 'tissued' and more nil by mouth. It had happened so many times before with no helpful effect. He was like a revolving door.

From the PSN

'I am a long term sufferer of Pancreatitis, (for the last seven years). I have no family local to myself other than my parents who are in their seventies

ANDREW'S STORY

*and in ill health themselves. So I constantly try
not to tell them just how bad things really are, I
don't want to worry them. As a result of this I have
had to deal with this completely on my own with
no help from anyone whatsoever. I cannot begin
to tell you how difficult the last seven years have
been. I have hit some real lows at times and if
someone would have handed me a loaded gun
when I was feeling so low I would gladly have
used it. I have spent seven years in 24 hour a
day, seven days a week pain. I'm unable to work;
I had to give up my store manager position with a
nationwide company and also consequently lost a
successful career in retail. As a result of losing
my job and my doctor's disbelief in my symptoms,
I couldn't get full benefits and our house was
repossessed because I couldn't pay the mortgage
repayments. I am now bankrupt. My eleven year
relationship has broken down and she has left with
my nine month old daughter, she is my only child
who I love very much. On the whole it's been
absolute hell on earth and the only thing that
keeps me going has been the thought of my
daughter. I look forward to seeing her so much.
The hardest part of all has been trying to contend
with all this absolutely alone, which is the reason
for this posting.*

*Now that I have found this site and become a
member it has been a real life saver. Just to know
that I am not the only one in this position and there*

are people out there who understand just how awful chronic Pancreatitis and all that goes with it really is. It has really helped me sitting down and reading everyone's problems and being able to relate to them. Things are not so bad for me and I can see light at the end of a very long tunnel and with continuing help from everyone at the PSN I feel life is worth living once again. Thank you all for just posting your letters and sharing your experiences on line, you have really helped this individual immensely.'

I felt the responsibility for Andrew was slowly being transferred to me, I couldn't abandon him he also was so alone. At least he had family and we would not let him down. I went to see Dr. Peter about it. He studied a spot on the wall just above my left shoulder. He said nothing and contributed nothing to the meeting. Each time I asked him a direct question hoping for an answer, he just shrugged his shoulders like a spoilt child. At least he didn't have his feet up on the desk as I had heard he did sometimes with other patients. It was impossible to get through to him and I left the surgery. He wasn't interested. Staff at the surgery were very distant and correct with me; there was no sign of friendliness or sympathy. Andrew felt he was being treated with no understanding whatsoever. He was just a nuisance or more.....

ANDREW'S STORY

From the PSN.

'I'm so glad I found this site as there are not many people around who understand this problem, especially the agony of it. I had my second big attack just over a week ago. The first was after I had my gallbladder removed and it took me by surprise. I'm told there is calcification somewhere in the pancreas and that there is little that can be done about it, does anyone know any different? The pain is incredible isn't it; the only description I can think of is thunderbolts and lightening, very, very frighteing! Does anyone feel like they're not always taken seriously when writhing around in agony in A&E? I saw the looks that said, oh no, not another abdoe pain trying for a fix! I did actually get morphine that last time, but the time before that, I was virtually ignored and made to feel that I was wasting their time and their precious resources. I'm a qualified nurse of twenty years and I was astounded. I'd like to think I treat my patients with more empathy than I experienced, I hope it is the exception to the rule! What have others experienced? I hope this finds you all well and pain free!'

And,

'Hi, you get used to the pain… I used to scream the place down with my first attacks as it felt like

my body was trying to rip itself inside out or something, but now I can feel that same pain and just look normal. You just get used to it and suffer in silence. You can turn up at the doctors and unless you are going ooh and ahhh, he thinks that you are not in pain!

My attacks have been less severe since I started taking Zoton. I was bringing up terrible bile and blood and suffering terrible heartburn during my attacks……'

And then,

'Chronic Pancreatitis, (My Personal Experience)

I am partially disabled with Chronic Pancreatitis. On my good days, I feel like I can move the world. On my bad days, I can't even move from bed.

Pancreatitis is a painful, often debilitating disease characterized by intense pain and digestive problems, sometimes accompanied by diabetes. The digestive problems demand that you can never be too close to the bathroom! People with Pancreatitis often look quite normal and healthy but have problems that can't been seen. No one can see the pain I'm in and no one can know that I have to deal with maybe as many as twelve bowel movements every day.

ANDREW'S STORY

*I first learnt about Pancreatitis in December 1995
when I was admitted to hospital with intense
abdominal pain. After a simple blood test I was
told I had Pancreatitis. It was severely inflamed
with multiple abscesses, two of which were the
size of grapefruits and severely infected. I had six
surgeries within two weeks and was given a one in
three chance of survival. I lost three stone in
weight. There were to be many complications
including infections.'*

I won't describe them all dear reader, it is
gruesome! I will give a shortened version of the
next few months for this patient.

*'I lost my home and many of my belongings,
Social Security had not been able to help me up to
this point and without my mum and dad my
address might have been, third box on the right, if
I was lucky, it might have been under a bridge.*

*A Celiac Plexus Block was tried for pain
management. Needles full of long lasting
anaesthetic are injected both sides of the spine, it
worked for only a few hours. My right thigh was
numb for several days! Because of the surgery
and scar tissue, it might prove impossible to get
the right spot!*

*Another CP Block three months later didn't work
either. The doctor tried Fentanyl patches, they*

drove me crazy the first day, it is such a powerful drug and irritated my skin so much it was difficult to wear them for the three days each patch is good for.

A year later, I saw a pain specialist and we dropped the patches. I am now taking methadone, the same drug given to heroin addicts but useful for pain reduction. (Do I remember something about liquid slugs?) *I'm also taking something for breakthrough pain. I have noticed that this tends to slow down my bowel movement, anyone else would be constipated, but this tends to make me almost normal, as long as I keep taking plenty of Creon.* (Digestive enzymes)

At last I have Disability Allowance, I had to go to appeal to decide if I was disabled or not. In all it took nearly three years. Thank goodness my parents gave me a place to stay and something to eat and drink during this time when I had nowhere else to go. It seems that government doesn't know about this disease either.

Four months later, my blood sugar has been on the high side from time to time, not severe but since I have little pancreas left, I would become a diabetic. The doctor said that pills will not help as they only stimulate the pancreas to produce more insulin and as I haven't got much pancreas left.....

ANDREW'S STORY

December 1999. I'm still taking methadone for pain. The doctor has increased the dose. So far I have managed to stay out of hospital though the daily pain seems to be getting worse. I'm watching my blood glucose levels as they seem to be creeping up, but so far so good!

June 2000. Nothing has changed much. I seem to have levelled off. I still deal with pain daily. I came close to going to A&E a few times but I know they will only give a shot of morphine and keep me in a ward 'nil by mouth' for a few days, then kick me out again when the pain subsides. That's about all they can do. If things get worse I have the option of more surgery.

November 2001. I lost my gastro doctor today. He has gone to greener pastures and I wish him well. I made a great first impression on him when I showed him my drain and promptly dumped a load of bile down the sink in his examination room! For that he said he will never forget me! I greatly fear strange new doctors, given what I have been through. It's comforting to find a doctor who knows about Pancreatitis and will talk to you about it, instead of rushing you out because he has another patient waiting.

I'm still taking methadone but it is not working nearly so well I think I am becoming tolerant of it.'

I drew this to the attention of Andrew and he read it. "It could be me', he said.

*   *   *

We took Andrew shopping which he loves to do. He bought some groceries and a t-shirt. Written on it in green florescent print was:

Your story has truly touched my heart.
Never before have I met anybody with so many
problems as you. You have my deepest
sympathy.
Now piss off and stop bothering me.

He was exhausted when we got back and I went to pick up Andrew's medication for him. He waited in the car; good days were getting less frequent. This time the pharmacist said I needed a letter from Andrew giving me permission to pick up the medication! I went to the car and brought Andrew back to the pharmacy counter and said to him, "Will you tell this man that you want me to pick up your medication for you?" He did and I said, "Go and sit down in the car and wait for me there."

The pharmacist carried on shuffling papers and looked at me, I said, "Can I have the medication then?" and he said, "Have you got it?" "Got what?" I said. "The letter." I said, "You heard Andrew tell you to give it to me." "Well, I can't file

ANDREW'S STORY

that can I?" I had to go and get Andrew from the car again to have the medication handed to him. Then he said, "I know your sort, look at all the doctors you've worn out, I've counted at least seven moves of practice." How did he have access to Andrew's notes? I dropped a note into Dr. Peter asking for an appointment to see him about this problem but never had an answer.

*   *   *

Back at Grove Park, the man who administered acupuncture was great. He was approachable and we could talk to him. At first there was no improvement but slowly there was a little relief for an hour or so. He was convinced that it would take time as the pain had a long history, but there was hope of more improvement. At first the appointments were every two weeks, then three and four weeks apart. We all stuck at it, me getting Andrew to the appointments and the acupuncturist sticking in the pins!

Andrew had always fought shy of baring his soul to anyone, he had too much experience of having to cover up how things really were because few believed him. He had to keep working and he had a wife who believed what the doctors told her, as we all did! With hindsight no one, it seems, was on Andrew's side during these middle years. It was difficult for him digging up what was very deeply hidden. The pain psychiatrist was patient and progress was being made, until he moved to a different job some 300 miles away!

The advertisement for the vacancy didn't attract any response first time but a second advert succeeded and a part time lady psychologist was appointed. We saw the pain doctor in between time and he joked that if Andrew wanted to retrain, he could think about psychology, "This is a £50,000 a year job being advertised and no takers," he said. We waited for a continuation appointment with the new lady but it didn't come. Another appointment came to see the pain doctor and he said he would write to her for an appointment. Nothing else changed, but this man always ended a session with "Don't forget. I'm always here for you." One day I asked him what he meant by that and he said, "Andrew can always ask to see me any time". He then said, "The problem is that he (Andrew) comes with baggage!" We were then swiftly shown out and I didn't get a chance to ask what did that mean! Another appointment: did not arrive in the post!

Eventually there was a letter from the secretary of the new lady psychologist saying, that due to reorganizing the department, Andrew would not be seen for a least a year, maybe eighteen months!

From the PSN

ANDREW'S STORY

'I have only been suffering with Chronic Idiopathic Pancreatitis since 2000. However, I am just worn out and have been quite down lately. I have enormous support from friends and family, I'm truly blessed by all of them. I am sick and tired of the physical symptoms, pain, nausea, vomiting and fatigue. But emotionally I'm feeling drained and alone. I feel like other Pancreatitis sufferers are the only ones who truly understand what I am going through and how horrible and miserable it is……..

I'm just feeling beat by this monster, will it every go away? I just want to get on with my life. I'm 28 and sometimes feel I will never be normal again. I find it hard to be committed and consistent with my job and it's hard to plan social outings because I just can never tell how I'll be feeling…I would welcome any encouragement I'm so frustrated with this Pancreatitis.'

In between all this Dr. Knight moved to the Bristol Royal Infirmary. Andrew was asked if he would like to see Dr. Knight there, or would he like to stay at the Weston Hospital as it wasn't so far to travel. Andrew was very sure he would go to Bristol if I would take him. I felt his mental health was beginning to wobble and Dr. Knight asked him to come and see him in his clinical research time for some psychological support. Dr. Knight was now head of research at the university laboratory and senior lecturer in health. He gave us his phone message service number and email address and said *'contact me anytime'*. His concern for Andrew's wellbeing was beyond what we could reasonably expect from anyone. Nothing was too much trouble.

He asked the local hospital to look after Andrew's day to day diabetes care, but they said they didn't have a pump service so they couldn't. They were about to set up such a service and would contact us when they could, but we never heard from them. The lady doctor from Bournemouth was now working at Grove Park. We were so happy that she had been appointed; we knew her reputation, now perhaps things might improve. I wrote to her saying how pleased we were that she had come to Taunton and I hoped she would be happy here. I asked did they have the software to print out Andrew's pump readings. Would it be possible to come in and use it? I never had any contact from her. Just the secretary phoned in response, she had been instructed to tell me NO! I wondered why the new doctor had reacted in that way. Who had been saying what to her? They might be upset with me, but that was no reason to withdraw treatment from Andrew. The pump is simply another way to deliver insulin. Day to day care of diabetes is nothing to do with a pump service

ANDREW'S STORY

Dr. Knight began to see Andrew monthly. If he wasn't well enough to travel he would give us an appointment for the next week and so on until we could get there. He asked what was happening about the pain treatment and we said well, not a lot, in fact, nothing really. What was happening about the gastro problems of vomiting, weight variation and mal-absorption, we were waiting for an appointment for a liver biopsy. What was happening about the psychotherapy, well nothing, we were still waiting for an appointment, and Andrew was smoking too much, it worried me. Dr. Knight said, "He has too many problems to deal with, we have to pick them off one at a time. Don't worry about the smoking when the others are under control we will worry about that!"

For me, it was very comforting to hear this as most people would tell me that, "Andrew was smoking far too much for his own good." What could I do about it? The sympathetic support I received from Dr. Knight was so very welcome, not too much of it about!

Eventually the GP said Andrew should have counselling. He would arrange it. A letter came inviting Andrew to make an appointment. Two weeks later I knew it wasn't done, did the doctor really think he was capable of sorting this out? I asked Andrew if he would like me to do it. I phoned on his behalf and was told the counsellor was on holiday, they would phone in a month. Six weeks later, nothing, and when I saw the GP he said, "He hasn't made contact with the counsellor you know." I said that I had, and in spite of being told they would contact me, nothing had happened. A quick change of attitude and he advised that I phone again. When Andrew did turn up for his appointment, he was told, "You should have been here last week." He didn't go again.

*   *   *

Our youngest son was now working full time and so far, he had never taken time off with sickness. He paced himself as best he could and was fortunate enough to keep his M.E. mostly under control. He would take it easy when he thought he was tired and rest instead of going out on the town with his friends. He decided that it was time for him to move into his own home, so while one son was giving up his home, the next was taking steps to own his first home. It was very exciting for him.

The house he settled on was five years old and in a small gated development, they said for security. I think it was because the local authority didn't want to adopt the road. There seems to be a move away from councils taking ownership of these small developments. I don't think there is any saving on council tax; the owners have to pay for street lighting, repairs, cleaning, maintenance and so on in their annual service charge.

Stephen's house is blessed with a garage, but not all of the houses have them, most have a parking space and there are only three parking spaces for visitors among thirty houses! Since he moved in, other small areas nearby have been built and some have no parking space at all. It's very short sighted of planners to allow this. The roads are already full of 'residents only' parking. What happened to the law which said all new housing units must have parking space? I'm sure I remember that. If it has been quietly dropped it is very silly. It causes so much stress to residents and it isn't necessary, it can be avoided. The roads seem not to be as wide as they were and it is so difficult to get through. If it is a way of traffic calming, it doesn't do anything for temper calming! Fortunately the house is close enough for Steve to walk to work; in fact it is quicker than getting the car out and driving in the rush hour traffic! He quite enjoys the leisurely exercise to work. He can entertain friends easier at his own home and we are not there to cramp his style!

Chapter 10

Bankrupt

The volunteer, who specialized in housing benefit matters at the CAB, was only in the office once a fortnight and my phone call had just missed her. I was away the next time she was there and Andrew forgot to phone her! Eventually we all caught up with each other and another housing benefits application form was filled in. This time the lady went with Andrew to the council office, she asked for a receipt from them and filed it in the CAB office file. Nothing was heard from the council and when I enquired what was happening to Andrew's housing benefit application, it could not be found, again.

I phoned CAB but the lady had moved out of the area and as yet had not been replaced! I explained on the phone that they had the receipt and was told, "No, it's up to the client to keep that, CAB doesn't keep it." After a long explanation she went to look and found it in the office file! When I produced it at the council office, they also found the application!

The Disability Rights Handbook published each year by the Disability Alliance is a mine of useful information on all aspects of disability. I first heard

ANDREW'S STORY

about it on a radio programme. Their advice is, always get a receipt for any correspondence from all authorities. This losing of forms and other documents must be standard practice for them to mention it!

I saw the customer services lady at the housing department who said that Andrew's form would be dealt with as soon as possible. I asked if they would need any documents from the sale of Andrew's flat and she said not.

A few days later, there was a phone call from the Council asking for some details of the flat sale. I passed the query on to Andrew and he said he would look for the answers. Several weeks later he still had not produced it and I went round to help him look for it. We took the paperwork into the office. Several weeks later they wanted more information. Where was the proof that we had lent him money? If I had known they would want proof I would have kept it, but as Andrew paid us what he owed, I threw away the paper work. That way I didn't get it muddled up with what was paid and what was not paid. With all the advice we had asked for, no one said I would have to prove what I had or had not lent him!

His money was running out again and people were beginning to chase him. The phone was cut off and the emergency Piper phone line sent back.

I thought we had an agreement with Piperline; they were to tell me if the BT bill wasn't paid and I would sort it out. We found one of the problems; they had the wrong telephone number! No wonder when I was away for four days and asked them to give him a wake up call, so he would get to a hospital appointment, they said he didn't answer! Who knows where it was ringing, it wasn't at his new flat. He did make it to hospital, I was so impressed, but then he said he hadn't slept at all that night so didn't need a wake up call!

He had told me before that often his mind was too full of pain signals so that he couldn't sleep. The body needs to be in sleep mode in order to fall asleep and if all your pain signals are saying ouch ouch, you can't sleep! Eventually exhaustion will take over and sleep will relieve the pain. It's not surprising that he doesn't always do things when he say's he will. He told me once that he must be related to a Spaniard, tomorrow, tomorrow....but in reality pain makes you tired and weary and life is hard to cope with.

The Piperline when activated would ring in the office and they would phone me to go round and see what the problem was. As Andrew had a mobile phone and could phone me away, we didn't have it re-installed. I was concerned that no one had told me the bill was not paid and that because the number was wrong, there was no warning that the line was to be disconnected! This should have rung alarm bells for me, but I believed Andrew when he said, everything was OK! 'Are you managing your finances and paying your bills, electric, water and so on', *'yes stop worrying'!*

I didn't know he had almost none of the money left from the sale of his flat and the bills were piling up again. He had also taken on paying the cost of the insulin pump sundries £800 per year; he said he could afford it!

*   *   *

The day of the DLA appeal came and we met up with Linda from DIAS at an office in the Department of Work and Pensions. We had sent some papers of what the disease was all about but there wasn't really much to say, except we thought the decision was wrong! I did have a photo copy of the 'out of hours' letter, which the doctor had sent to me. Linda said it was good evidence of Andrew's condition and gave it in as a late submission.

We waited for our turn with Andrew running off to the toilet to either be sick or sit down every few minutes. Our turn came and we went in to the board room. There were three people on the panel, one of whom was a doctor. We explained why we had appealed and then each person on

the panel asked Andrew questions about his illness, how long he had had it, how it affected his everyday life. The doctor looked at the list of medication and said. "I would have expected you to be on replacement enzymes if you have no pancreas." Andrew looked at the list and said, "I am taking Creon, it's the last one on the list." "Oh yes,'" he said, "I didn't see it there!"

The lady on the panel, I think she had a background in Social Services, asked her questions. Sometimes I know it hurt Andrew to answer and I did so want to answer for him, but knew I couldn't. At one point she asked something and I said I could answer if she wanted me to, but she put her hand up and I had to leave it to him. It was very personal and sometimes he didn't want to say, but he struggled with the answers and the words eventually came out. How many young men want to tell you how often they mess their pants?

He also explained that sometimes he was very sick and couldn't get out of bed and on occasions didn't make it to the toilet. They asked what he would do on a good day and he said that if he went into town shopping, he would navigate round by where each toilet was. He knew where they were in each shop or area that he was in. He found it very embarrassing to admit he could be taken short and to explain what happened when he was. He said he was very young and it was all too embarrassing to deal with.

In particular Andrew said that the smell made him want to be alone and hide away. He told them that his specialist asked if the steatorrhoea was offensive and he said it certainly was. I'm sure that was one of the problems at his last place of employment. I could just imagine the reaction of some less sympathetic colleagues, 'Core blimey, who's done it this time, you trying to gas us out!'

The hearing was over very quickly, or it seemed that way, and we prepared to go home expecting to hear the result in a week or two. We were shown back into the waiting room and the young man who was looking after us said he thought the panel were going to make a decision now and we should wait. He came back into the room with the decision; Andrew had been awarded top rate for mobility and middle rate for care! We didn't really expect to win and we were delighted. Linda was not surprised she said we had a very good case.

We phoned home with the news and then asked our advocate if we could take her out for a little light lunch. Like Andrew she was tee total but was happy to accept a soft drink and sandwich in celebration.

All this time Andrew had been living on incapacity benefit and eventually income support, and nothing else apart from the money left from the sale of the flat!

On the way home we called in to the pharmacy for his medication again. This time in front of a shop full of people the pharmacist said to me, "Back for more"' "'I don't know what you mean," I said, "I just wanted to pick up Andrew's prescription." On a piece of paper the pharmacist had written the number of pills Andrew should have had over a given time and how many he actually had! "I expect you put him up to asking for more than he needs," he said. I asked, "Why I would do that." "I expect you sell them on the street corner," was the answer in a very loud voice as he passed the medication to me! I was very angry but Andrew asked me not to complain as he said, "I have to go back there again whether I like it or not!" I thought what was prescribed was a matter between the GP and patient, apparently I was wrong. Mr. Green now works for the PCT and has quite a prestigious job!

I wrote to the pain department telling them what happened and asking them to get the pain under better control and help Dr. Peter to manage it better, but nothing happened.

ANDREW'S STORY

From the PSN. Advice was being sought on the subject of the DLA, this was one answer.

'Please do not just accept what you have been told by the DSS. My husband was totally housebound and unable to even get out of bed for nearly a year and yet he was told he didn't qualify. We had to fight extremely hard and appeal against decisions, but eventually he was given Disability Benefit and also Severe Disability Allowance.

The claim forms concerned do not seem to have any real relevance to CP/TP (chronic Pancreatitis/total pancreatectomy) sufferers, as they concentrate on whether or not you have all your limbs, whether or not you can go to the loo by yourself, whether you can dress yourself and whether you can lift a saucepan. I found it easier to complete the forms in as much detail as possible and then to send an accompanying letter explaining in detail, why and how this disease affects your life. Our GP also gave us a letter which was very helpful.

I am absolutely positive that the DSS makes the claims procedure as long, painful and demoralising as possible, in order to deter people from claiming. It took three appeals for us, but after nine months, my husband's claim was allowed and back dated.

My advice would be not to take no for an answer and to keep appealing until someone listens!

Good luck and best wishes.'

On occasions Andrew found the walk to the doctor's surgery to pick up his medication too much, although he had worked out where he could rest and have a cigarette on route. There were no village seats but there were low stone walls around the churchyard and a flight of steps that were useful for resting on. He would phone sometimes and ask if I would pick up his prescription for him. This time when I got to his flat I found he couldn't move for pain, again, he was dehydrated and very poorly. He didn't look as though he had washed for several days. I called the Ambulance and he was taken in to hospital, again.

Now I could go into his bathroom and kitchen which is something he had managed to manoeuvre me out of by some means or other for a few weeks now. It was a health hazard! I don't think he had managed to clean up for sometime and he had often not made it to the toilet to be sick! In the kitchen there was half finished food from take-a-way shops, home delivery service and refuse sacks which had not been put out for some weeks. On closer inspection the smell came from the rotting food. There were rotting fruit and

ANDREW'S STORY

vegetables which hadn't been taken out of the bags they were sold in. The refrigerator needed a good clean and the milk was off, but I'm not sure the cooker had been used; it didn't need cleaning at all!

I phoned Social Services again, saying that he was in hospital; I said I didn't mind cleaning the flat but I did want them to see the state of it first as it was a health hazard. The young lady said she took my word for that and if I would clean up she would find a way to help matters if she could. She was as good as her word and phoned back saying as he was in hospital he was entitled to a 'discharge package' and she had put in place an hour a week domestic help plan.

There were six washing machine loads of clothes, sheets and so on and it took me all the week that he was in hospital, to get the flat back into order. On his return I asked why he hadn't asked for help before it got into such a state and he said, "I kept hoping I would feel better and be able to do it myself. I didn't want you to have to do it all."

Sarah from Social Services came to see Andrew and went over what had been happening to him. She was the only one I had met who said she had another client with Pancreatitis! That was interesting and I asked her how it affected him, she said, "Much the same as Andrew really, in and out of hospital all the time with uncontrollable pain and often sick." Many years ago we had asked if there was anyone in the area with this disease who we could meet and talk to and although we were always told there were others, we were never put in touch with anyone. I had often wondered if in fact there was anyone else.

Although one hour a week wasn't much, it was a help and it was also someone else going in to see he was OK. She could keep the kitchen and toilet reasonable in that time and with sickness and steatorrhoea that was a great help. He liked his clothes to be ironed, as he said, "Pride in my appearance is all I have left." But ironing aggravated his back ache, leaning over at that angle. Cleaning lower levels was also difficult.

The same lady usually came and was kind and efficient, but occasionally a different person was sent, sometimes they didn't arrive at all! Once when I phoned the office to say that no one came that day, they said, "Sometimes our older clients say that the home help didn't come and the girls occasionally say that the client's memory is not good and they have been! Andrew is young enough to know if they came or not." Soon after that a book was provided and the 'girls' wrote a brief account of what they had done on a visit then both parties signed and dated the book.

ANDREW'S STORY

Sarah asked an Occupational Therapist to visit Andrew to see if there was anything that could be adapted to help him. He explained that it was difficult to get in and out of the bath because of the back pain and because the stomach muscles had been cut, the strength to lift himself wasn't there. As a temporary measure, she got him a bath seat so that he didn't have such a long way to raise himself, and then said, "I think we should apply for a shower fitting for you," to which Andrew agreed as it was much easier to shower than to bath. Sometimes he would use our shower when he came to us.

The plans were drawn up and a grant agreed with the Council, all Andrew had to do was obtain three quotations. Just doing that seemed more than he could cope with. I didn't think I should do it for him, I didn't want anyone to think I had 'put him up to it', so that I would get 'a free shower installed in my flat!' A couple of months later when I asked what was happening he said he didn't know who to ask, so we went through Yellow Pages and found some names to phone. He didn't phone and never did get the quotations to send to the Council.

The housing benefit department were still asking for more information, each time going further and further back into our affairs. Much of the information they were asking for we simply didn't have anymore. Eventually they asked to see our bank statements and other information personal to us, not Andrew. It was not us making the application for housing benefit! If we didn't comply it would be assumed that we had something to hide! So we sent our accounts, bank statements, invoices and utility bills, in fact everything. I thought it was a bit of a cheek really.

*   *   *

Surfing the net I came across EuroPac. It is a European research project centred in Manchester for the UK and they have links with Liverpool. They are interested particularly in Childhood Hereditary Pancreatitis which I had never heard of. I asked Andrew if he was interested in pursuing this and he said he was. I contacted them and they phoned back immediately. Andrew was fifteen when the disease first started and he just qualified for investigation as to whether it might be childhood hereditary Pancreatitis. The doctor said they had traced about 300 families, some with children as young as two! The poor souls, how they and their parents coped I can't begin to imagine, I guess like us, they had no other choice.

EuroPac and I exchanged emails and I was asked if we would mind a copy of our details being sent to Liverpool, we had no problem with that. Then we were contacted by one of the Liverpool team and asked if we would like to come up and see them! Not that they could promise anything useful, what an opportunity to be invited to one of the top centres of excellence! Professor Neoptolemus wanted to see Andrew's x-rays and I arranged for them to be sent by Grove Park. I also asked for a copy of the operation notes to send and I was changed £17 for them! We had to have a referral, Andrew asked the GP and he said yes! The appointment arrived and on the appointed day we took the train to Liverpool.

Our appointment was 2pm and we thought that was plenty of time to get our train back to the West Country. At 3.30 we had still not been seen and Andrew was uncomfortable with sitting and it was hot, he always did drink a lot and his water bottles were empty. He went in search of somewhere to refill them. I was worried he would miss his turn but he didn't. At 4.15pm we were shown in and the doctor didn't seem all that pleased to see us. He looked at the x-rays that had been sent and asked a lot of questions, then said he didn't think Andrew had a spleen, to which Andrew said he thought he did! If the spleen has been removed then antibiotic injections are needed on a regular basis.

He quizzed Andrew as to why he was on pain medication when he had had the total

Pancreatectomy. What about the methadone, was he still on it? Andrew said, "I have been off that for years," and we both looked at each other. The only remark as we left was, "You could be offered a BITS operation, to sever the nerves in the chest which might help with the pain, but I don't do it for people who are still taking pain medication!" We left, we missed our train back, fortunately there was another one, but it was a slow train and stopped everywhere it seemed. It was 12.30am when we got back, deflated, and I wondered why I had put Andrew through all that exhausting day for, I didn't think we had achieved anything.

At the PSN they said some people do have that experience with this man, but some had found Liverpool very helpful. I guess our faces didn't fit, but no, we were told, he just didn't like people on pain medication! So what is someone with the same sort of pain experienced by cancer sufferers to do, suffer in silence? Later some one on the PSN board referred to this man as 'a cocky little blighter'. That just about summed it up; brilliant I'm sure, but cocky. It took Andrew days to get over the effort and journey. The train fare was £134, for what?

I emailed the Professor and said,

ANDREW'S STORY

'Your first question threw us a bit; you emailed us and invited us to make an appointment, what made you think it was a self referral? There were so many things we wanted to ask you, it's a pity we spent so long on the methadone thing, we didn't tell you about it, who did? Did they tell you it was prescribed and after the operation he got off it on his own? How can swollen ankles, which have been occurring occasionally since well before he became a diabetic and before the total Pancreatectomy, be caused by nutritional issues? I don't understand, can you explain? What can we do about it?

My younger son suffers from M.E. He knows how lucky he is that it is now recognised and he is not thought of as a malingerer, as did happen not so long ago. Also, my daughter has just been diagnosed with endometriosis after complaining of pain for twenty years.

A doctor friend of mine told me that some of his colleagues, who can't explain, play the blame game! I hope you find the time to read this and answer just some of our concerns. Andrew was very upset when we got home thinking he is being told it is all in his head, again!'

There was no answer! We never heard from him again.

Back at EuroPac, they said that as Andrew was adopted they couldn't do the blood tests and so on, but from their experience it was 99% certain that his Pancreatitis was hereditary.

*   *   *

Ron and I decided that we would take a week's holiday. With Social Services weekly visit to Andrew, him feeling better and Steve promising to keep in touch with Andrew, we thought we had it all covered as best we could. So off we went on a National Trust holiday up the River Rhine and Moselle.

Oh the freedom of not thinking whether I should visit. But tempered with, 'I wonder what's going on!' No point in phoning Andrew on his mobile, it seems as though he has an allergy to it and has given up answering the phone. Steve says he is OK though and if he isn't he can call the ambulance himself, he's done it before.

We had never been river cruising before. We flew from Bristol, so much better than the four hour journey to Gatwick. Our trip started with an accompanied cruise round the Amsterdam canals. I had never been there but Ron had when he toured with the National Theatre. We passed the Anne Frank Museum and there were still long queues to go in at three in the afternoon. I know

ANDREW'S STORY

that Amsterdam has the title of the Venice of the North but I couldn't see it myself. It had a lot of water, yes, charm of its own, yes, but Venice, I'm not so sure. There were many houseboats and I remembered when we first got married that I had wanted to look at a houseboat for sale on the Thames, but I was told, "I'm not living in a damp place like that!"

We started out of Amsterdam for Cologne and I was soon captivated by the landscapes we were passing. So many pretty villages, towns and castles, it really was magical. I could let my imagination run wild and see Rhine maidens everywhere! At night with everything lit up, it looked like fairly land! It was stunning! Northern European towns, German ones in particular, are noted for their cleanliness.

We passed the Lorelei Rock. It was different to what I expected but I don't know what I did expect really! On the way home we stopped at Arnhem with all the war time connotations. The 'Bridge' was just a little way from where we moored and I found it rather moving to stand and look at the now peaceful scene and remember the films I had seen about it. My father was 'in the war' but he came home to us safely and with lots of stories. Thankfully none like that! The next day we visited the House and Garden of Het Loo and then we were home! It was all over so quickly, but we felt we had to be back.

He was OK and survived our absence! We said we would take him shopping the next day as his stores were a bit low and a trip to the supermarket would be good. The local village shops were fine but sometimes the town was nice to visit for a change.

We arranged that I would call on Andrew the next day, I arrived and let myself in and he wasn't up, nothing too unusual about that. He slept longer and longer so I woke him up and waited. There was a letter on the front door mat. It seemed the bailiff had called but the letter said he was out! Andrew said he didn't know what it was all about and I explained that bailiffs don't call without reason or warning. As I bent down to pick up the keys I had just dropped, I saw something under the settee and pulled it out. It was an unopened letter and as I looked there were more. There were more down the back of the settee, under the cushions, under the coffee table at the end of the settee; in all there were 56 unopened letters.

The bailiff had come from the council, they wanted their council tax. I phoned and said, "We have been through this, you were going to sort this out with 'One' at the job centre." 'One' is a system, by which all advice on benefits is centred in one

ANDREW'S STORY

place, the Job Centre. They told Andrew many months before that he shouldn't be paying council Tax, he should be entitled to council tax benefit. We had written to the Council and they said they would look into it. As we had heard no more and having no experience in these matters, we thought it was taken care of. The council said they would stop the bailiff calling and sort it all out. The following week, another letter through the door saying the bailiff had called but you were out! I phoned the Council again and the following week the same thing happened again! I wrote to the chief executive and we got a letter saying it would be dealt with. We didn't have the bailiff on the door step again, however, as no council tax benefit had been agreed, he did owe the money!

Andrew wanted to go shopping and said he would open the letters later. On the way back to his home he asked if I would stop at the surgery and pick up his prescription. When we got there I asked if he would like me to go in for it and he said yes he would wait in the car. No problem this time but I had to sign a sheet of A4 paper which had been prepared saying that I had taken the medication away on behalf of Andrew.

When we got back he said he was too tired to deal with the letters now. The next day it was the same thing and in the end I had to insist on helping him with opening them saying, we will throw away the

ones that are just advertising and the pile will go down. He stopped prevaricating and we opened them all. Most were asking for, or demanding money. I think he was just plain frightened to open them and hoped they would go away, but they didn't.
Now it seems, he had an allergy to answering the phone and opening letters!

Among all the letters I noticed one on the coffee table to us, it was saying goodbye and he hoped we would forgive him. When I asked what it was all about he said, "Oh, I thought I had thrown that away, I was very down the other week and thought about ending it all, but I thought better of it. I'm OK now." I believed him but later he confessed to the psychiatrist, in front of me, that he had taken an overdose and was disappointed that he just woke up again!

I asked Social Services for help but Sarah had moved on. I was told that they would find a support worker but nothing happened. I asked CAB to assist him and so began a long hard job for them sorting out his finances. They decided that the best way forward was to declare Andrew bankrupt and I lent him the £250 needed for the court expenses. This was before the DLA appeal.

Still no news from the housing benefits office. It seemed to me they kept moving the goal posts!

ANDREW'S STORY

Each time we thought we had satisfied them, they wanted more information. Eventually the council made Andrew's housing benefit application 'deficient'. I had not heard this term used in that way and didn't know what it meant. Enquiries made it clear; it is frozen, not closed and not determined. They say there is not enough information to make a decision and so it is left on the shelf, there can be no appeal and no further application.

Chapter 11

Disability or Age Discrimination?

Andrew could not pay his rent and we found ourselves in the position of having to take steps to obtain possession of the flat so that we could either sell it or rent it out again, in order to pay the mortgage on our house. We had to make our own son homeless as no housing benefit was going to be paid.

Through the window of Andrew's flat I saw someone I knew walking to the village. She had come out of one of the Council's one bedroom sheltered bungalows near by. Later I saw her again, she said she had moved and was very happy having sold her cottage; it was too big for her now. Although a little older than me she was fit and well. Then I met someone else I knew who also had just moved to sheltered accommodation! Again there seemed nothing wrong with him as far as I knew, he was a retired post man who spent all his spare time photographing local wild life! He was a very popular local character and often in demand to give talks and slide shows. I suggested to Andrew that we ask for sheltered housing for him as it would be good for there to be someone on call if he had a problem and was in trouble. He thought that was a good idea and asked me to do it.

We contacted the Council and said that Andrew had to move as he couldn't pay his rent and could he be considered for sheltered housing. We were told there is no sheltered accommodation for people under 60, try Social Services! Social Services said we don't have any housing stock, the Council have houses, what are they talking about, go back to them! I phoned back the Council and told them what Social Services had said.

Eventually they sent a homelessness officer to interview Andrew and he wanted me to be with him. The officer explained the difference between general needs accommodation, sheltered accommodation of which there was none for under 60's and the obligations on the Council as far as homelessness was concerned. It was very complicated and I found it hard to grasp all at once. Andrew had given up trying to follow the conversation and simply slumped in the chair! I asked, "If there is no sheltered housing for under 60's, isn't that discrimination?" The question was ignored! She asked lots of questions and in particular wanted to know about his illness. It's very difficult to tell people in a short time how it affects him. The affects are very dramatic so you have to be careful not to let them think you are exaggerating. That's difficult! He had lost the thread of all the questions and left it to me to answer for him. Eventually she asked him to sign a form to give her permission to enquire about which benefits he was on and said she would be in touch. It is a bit of a maze trying to understand the policies of the housing department. My head was spinning and Andrew had just given up.

A long time after and with help from the Information Officer, we read her office notes which said, he looked very well and smoked continuously, mother did all the talking.

From the PSN

'Outwardly we do appear to be well although inwardly we are gritting our teeth and trying to put up with varying degrees of pain. If I push myself I can go for a walk and distract myself but the pain is ever present even though I am not suffering an attack at the moment. Interestingly the GP I saw last time I had an acute attack just told me to avoid fatty food and go home! No medication or diagnosis given, except it must be my gallbladder. He missed the point completely, as I told him, I was unable to sleep, vomiting every time I took a bite or a sip of something and doubled over with abdominal pain day and night. I told him all this but he must have thought I looked reasonably well nonetheless!'

ANDREW'S STORY

And

'This is a feature of Pancreatitis….. to be looking well while we are being torn to pieces by the pain inside us.'

I was talking to a friend about Andrew and she said she thought he would benefit from a (CPN) community psychiatric nurse. I didn't know there were such people but she said to ask his social worker. I did but Sarah had left and in her place was Trish. I explained the problems and she said she could refer him to a CPN. It was time for his annual assessment review, she would make an appointment to come out and see him. New to us she was friendly, sympathetic and spent sometime with Andrew talking to him and asking questions.

The result of her visit was a letter to say that he no longer qualified for domestic help and it was being withdrawn; he should use his DLA and organize it himself. She could not refer him to the CPN, if he felt he needed that service he should see his GP and as Andrew had no needs, she was closing his file! Great!

I wrote back and asked why he no longer qualified for help and why she couldn't refer him to the CPN when she had said she could? He did have needs and she should reopen his file! I said he used his

DLA to pay his rent and keep a roof over his head. A roof over your head is an important need for a disabled person. Would she also please tell the Occupational Therapist that as Andrew would have to move there was no need for the shower to be fitted? He needed help with finding another roof over his head and what could she do to help? Nothing happened!

Her attitude had changed and I wondered why. Had she spoken to the doctor and what had he said? Andrew would not go back to his GP so no request for a community psychiatric nurse, no help, or any input from Social services at all!

Eventually Trish said she was mistaken in her role and thought she could refer him to a CPN but had been told that she couldn't, she didn't say by whom. She would refer him for support from one of their agencies. It was their job to encourage Andrew to get up and dress, cook and clean for himself, and organize his life better. There had been a change of policy and domestic help was no longer provided. As social services would not be involved in that, she would close his file, again!

We asked to see Andrew's social services file. First being told that all third parties must be asked if they would mind us seeing it! I asked what happened if they did object, in that case we would not be able to see any of the letters. If the author objected there was no appeal. Fortunately there were no objections and an appointment was made to go to County Hall to read it. But come the day Andrew wasn't well enough and we postponed. Later we went to the social service office to see the file. There was very little in it and really nothing of interest. We wanted to know if there were any letters from the GP which might have changed Trish's attitude, but there was nothing, just a few letters of no consequence....

When I had been phoning Housing Associations, one had said, "We may be able to offer your son a support worker to help him maintain his tenancy." Anything was welcome and the system put in place, it took a little while but eventually Andrew had the services of Amanda. She worked with Andrew to see what could be done about his housing situation. Chronic constant pain dominates your life, saps energy and makes it difficult to do anything for long. With the other problems thrown in for good measure, he found it difficult to concentrate or find the will to do anything very much, but Amanda continues her visits which Andrew looked forward to. She was the only person apart from family and medics that he had much contact with.

The interim report from the council homelessness department came and it said that Andrew's case had been looked into and he was not 'medically vulnerable'. Therefore, he could not be housed as a homeless medically vulnerable person. I asked who said he was not medically vulnerable, had advice been taken? She told me that Dr. Morkane, the Director of Public Health at the Primary Care Trust had been asked if my son's disabilities would make him vulnerable and it was Dr. Morkane's opinion that it would not.

I emailed her and said,

'I guess I should ask what information did you give to Dr. Morkane? To be precise and accurate it is this:

Andrew had his first attack at fifteen. It became a chronic condition and at seventeen he had a partial Pancreatectomy to stop the pain. It didn't and when the pancreas stopped working altogether he had a Whipples operation which included a total Pancreatectomy. This did not stop the pain and he is now prescribed the sort of pain drugs that cancer patients use. We now know there is a 50% failure rate with this operation.

Andrew now has no natural insulin unlike most diabetics, who need to top up the amount of insulin in their body. He is a brittle diabetic with difficult management problems. His insulin is delivered by a pump which carries on working while Andrew has a bad pain day, can't eat or

ANDREW'S STORY

*keep food down and goes back to bed and sleeps
a lot. Usually it is very important for diabetics to
keep eating to keep a balance of insulin to food.
This is why he has a pump and is treated in
Bristol. His blackouts are more under control with
the pump.*

*Due to having his pancreas removed, he produces
no Pancreatic enzymes and must take enzymes to
digest food each time he eats. This causes weight
problems, last Christmas he lost three stones in
almost as many weeks. After treatment in Bristol,
he has regained almost all of it, but it is difficult to
maintain weight, which in turn affects diabetes.*

*He also has bacterial overgrowth, steatorrhoea
and balanitis.*

*The biggest problems of all are the results of
taking very strong pain killers and the depression
all this has brought upon Andrew.*

*On the whole Andrew manages to be very
independent with a little help from us when
needed; he has been awarded DLA at the top rate
for five years. He can't work.*

*If this does not make him a vulnerable person who
can I appeal to?*

Did you make it clear to Dr. Morkane what Andrew's problems are, (did I make it clear to you? We do not like to dwell on his problems too much, Andrew has to stay positive), can the report be re-submitted? I doubt whether Dr. Morkane has ever come across Childhood Pancreatitis before.

Thanks for your help.'

I asked her to confirm with Dr Morkane that he had made a correct judgement as I couldn't see how anyone with these major health problems could not be considered anything other than medically vulnerable. She said she would talk to Dr. Morkane again and in the meantime I wrote to the doctor asking if he had consulted Andrew's specialists.

Dr. Morkane phoned me, no he said, he had not spoken to specialists, he had asked the person who knew Andrew's medical history best, the GP and that was his advice! I said Andrew had not been registered with him for long, only about a year. His specialists had known Andrew much longer as he had been ill since he was fifteen years old. He then said a curious thing, "Aren't you the lady who wanted an insulin pump? I remember you." He promised to look at the advice again, and write to me. In a letter he said, "There were more important things to consider than his medical vulnerability," he didn't change his mind! We never told what these more important things were.

We had been on a coach outing with the National Trust and Andrew had come with us. It proved to be a bad day for him in many ways, bad pain, bad sickness, he had held up the coach from its departure time being in the toilet. So when we got home we went straight to the doctors to see if Andrew could have an injection of metoclopramide to stop the vomiting. We saw one of the partners who was a bit more sympathetic than some and as we waited for the injection to be prepared, we told her about our request for sheltered housing. She thought it would be good for him and later we phoned to ask if she would accept Andrew on to her books as he didn't really feel comfortable with Dr. Peter any more. "'I don't think I could do that," she said, "He wouldn't like it. None of us are allowed to see Andrew unless Dr. Peter isn't on duty. He thinks Andrew is avoiding him." He was right!

Astonishingly, when the final report arrived it said Andrew didn't fulfil the criteria of medical vulnerability. There was to be no help from the Council, as far as they were concerned, he could be homeless and live on the streets 'without detriment'. I spoke to one of Andrew's specialists who said, "That's ridiculous, just a look at his medication list would tell anyone that he is vulnerable!" He wrote a 'To whom it may concern' letter supporting Andrew's application. Another doctor said, "He cannot keep needles clean and insulin in a fridge if living on the streets," he also wrote a letter of support.

We asked for the report to be looked at again and in spite of the letters, which the housing department said, 'didn't tell them anything new', the report was upheld. What this means is that there are people living in sheltered housing who don't need it, they are fit and healthy, and there are young people with major health problems, living on the streets with no help at all, they are homeless! I seem to remember reading somewhere that people were encouraged to join up in the First World War, to create a land fit for heroes! Well they didn't get much justice then and nothing seems to have changed!

Amanda said, "If Andrew is not medically vulnerable he would qualify as homeless and he could apply for a place in a homeless person's hostel, let's make an appointment and see what they say." Amanda had worked at the hostel previously and I think she knew what they would say! All three of us went to the interview and having read the report the director of the hostel said, "Andrew, this is nothing against you, I'm sure you are a very nice young man but we couldn't have you here with a medication list like this, you would be a target, you are medically vulnerable and we can't house you! I'm very sorry. We would recommend that you go to Shelter for advice; would you like us to make an appointment?"

They made the phone call and we had an appointment for that afternoon! Amanda couldn't come as she had another appointment but she asked us to let her know what happened.

The first thing that Shelter said was, "Oh, they are still using that form, we asked the council to change it over a year ago and they said they would, it is not appropriate, but here it is again." He then read the report and said, "Housing reports like this can be challenged on three points of law and this report can be challenged on all three! It must be challenged in Court and it is time limited, so you have three days left to make a challenge if you want to. We can organize a solicitor if you wish." Andrew said he would like to challenge it and John left the room to make a phone call to the solicitor.

After he had left the room Andrew said, "I know him from school, if I had known I would be seen by someone I knew, I wouldn't have come." I told him we didn't have to go on with this; we could go home now if he wanted to but he said, "He knows now, it's too late."

John came back into the room and said, "Andrew, don't I know you from school?" "Yes," he said, "If you would prefer someone else who doesn't know you to look after your case, I can arrange that." It was very thoughtful of him to understand that Andrew might be embarrassed, but Andrew said it was OK. John then said that where a person is covered by the Disability Discrimination Act, that person is considered to be medically vulnerable in terms of housing! Diabetes is covered by that act. I told him about the Employment Tribunal and the Disability Rights Commission; I hadn't realised that it covered housing issues too.

He gave us a copy of the Homelessness Code of Guidelines of Vulnerability from the web site of the Office of the Duty Prime Minister,

8.13 states that the 'critical test' in connection with vulnerability is:

'Whether, when homeless, the applicant would be less able to fend for himself than an ordinary homeless person so that he would be likely to suffer injury or detriment, in circumstances where a less vulnerable person would be able to cope without harmful effects'.

ANDREW'S STORY

Code 8.15 says, 'housing authorities should have regard to any medical advice or social services advice obtainable, but the final decision on the question of vulnerability will rest with the housing authority. In considering whether such applicants are vulnerable, factors that a housing authority may wish to take in to account are:

1. The nature and extent of the illness and disability which may render the applicant vulnerable; and

2. The relationship between the illness or disability and the individual's housing difficulties.'

Code 8.17 say's, 'Physical disability or long term acute illness, such as those defined by the Disability Discrimination Act 1995 which impinge on the applicant's housing situation and give rise to vulnerability may be readily discernable, but advice from health or social staff should be sought, wherever necessary. As for all homelessness applications, the decision rests with the housing authority.'

It seems to me that the illness is destroying everything in Andrew's life making him very vulnerable! Surely they must be able to see that!

We saw the solicitor the next morning and his opinion was the same as John's, this report can be challenged on three points of law. Would Andrew like him to take on the case, legal aid would probably be available on application, "Definitely, please go ahead," said Andrew. "I must prepare our challenge and lodge it in court this afternoon." A barrister's opinion was obtained. He reviewed the case and concluded it had a high chance of success.

The case preparation continued and Taunton Deane began to send 'without prejudice' letters to the solicitor, a sign he thought that they may not let the case get as far as Court.

In the mean time I had contacted PALS, the Patient Advice and Liaison Service. I knew there was one at the hospital, but I haven't realised the Primary Care Trust also had one. I told her what had happened and asked why had the Director of Public Health told Taunton Deane that Andrew was not medically vulnerable? She said she would look into it and contact me…

*   *   *

Gail from Headway, social services agent, made an appointment to visit Andrew; she explained her role and gave him their handbook. He was pretty poorly when they met so after a little while she left. I cancelled her next visit as he was no better, there was no way in which he could get up and go shopping, then come home and do cooking and cleaning! He didn't improve and to save me the constant backwards and forwards to him, we brought him home to stay for a while. Several weeks later and with Christmas almost here, Andrew asked if he could stay with us until after the holiday as he didn't want to go home and be on his own at Christmas. Although it had already been arranged he would come to us for the days he wanted to sleep here. His two siblings were coming home and he was looking forward to being with them. It seemed quite like old times to have them all home again. The pain, vomiting and steatorrhoea did not let up.

Just before Christmas the PALS officer from the PCT phoned asking where Andrew was. She wanted to see him but didn't know where to contact him! I explained he was staying with us as he was not well and she arranged to come to our house to meet him. She brought the Director of Public Health with her! He was from the Antipodes somewhere but I didn't ask where. They were late, arriving at 4.20pm for a 4pm appointment and then at 4.50pm said, they must go as they had another meeting to attend, it was Friday afternoon! She said, "I can see he is far from well, we will try to arrange a case meeting with those involved with his care." I still didn't get an answer to why the PCT said Andrew was not medically vulnerable! Christmas came and went;

he was the only one I knew who lost weight over the festive period!

Eventually Ron and I agreed that no one was going to help Andrew and we had to do something about the flat, our savings were going down every month with mortgage repayments. Although Andrew paid what he could, the DLA didn't cover the rent/mortgage repayments.

We didn't want to live 'on family' with him as when he was poorly he sometimes didn't sleep at all and had the TV on most of the time. That would drive us mad, but if it was the way he could cope, we couldn't complain. Neither of us would like to have to deal with his continued problems on a daily basis! There was a need for him to have a part of the house to himself, even if it only gave him the peace of mind to know that he wasn't inflicting the stench of steatorrhoea on us. It was agreed with Andrew that he should move back home with us permanently. What a prospect for him as well as us! But as he said, "I do need someone near to call on when I'm in trouble." He was pleased that the problem of a roof over his head, which he could not see away out of, was being solved for him....

*   *   *

ANDREW'S STORY

Just as Ron was thinking about retiring, he had been asked to make a Double Bass. He looked at his records and calculated that he had made forty nine basses over the years. Thinking that fifty would be a good number to retire on, he carried on working for several months more and bass number fifty left the workshop for the Bournemouth Sinfonietta. Thanks to the accountants, the orchestra doesn't exist now! Who needs live musicians?

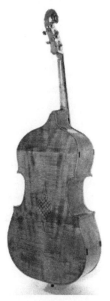

Many of the possessions left from a working life were in two store rooms over the main workshop and after Christmas we set to and cleared the rooms that had been used for storage for over thirty years. We thought the two rooms would make a self contained area for him. There is a separate entrance he could use for his front door.

The rooms were full of wood and all sorts of things needed for work. We hadn't got round to disposing of them yet, but we didn't want to throw them away. Wood for instrument making is expensive to buy but not readily disposable as it is very specialised being prepared by quarter sawing. There were blocks of wood for carving necks and scrolls and pegs for tuning smaller instruments and 'tuners' for basses. And so many bottles of resins to make varnishes, and stains for matching colours for instruments in for repair. All sorts of vessels were kept for mixing colours, and polishes of different kinds for different jobs. In fact the two rooms were completely full and it was difficult to open the door to get into them!

On book shelves in the store room, from floor to ceiling, there were consecutive years of model magazines, model engineering books, kite making books, text books of all kinds and dozens of plans. Our specialist books on violinmaking and makers were kept down stairs. They are sought after and very expensive to buy! Having given away some model aeroplanes and with a heavy heart, Ron took fifteen models that he had made, into the garden and burnt them. There was nowhere to keep them, it still left him twenty five in the loft, but that wasn't the point.

In the room behind was the half size violin made for April by Ron, kept in a beautifully veneered box made by my father. There was also a Chamber Bass which April had used in the National Youth Orchestra, two guitars and two trombones, leftovers from the boy's childhood. There were many other instruments including some 'early instruments made by Ron and a rebec we brought home from a holiday in North Africa. We had been on a working cruise which was great, the only way we would ever get such a holiday! The band had to work in the bar in the evening, they didn't get paid but wives went free, the musicians union soon put a stop to that. The piece de resistance of the instrument collection was half a violin, cut in half lengthways! (Just a cheap mass produced one)! It was to show people what a violin looked like on the inside and what made it work! Ron used this from time to time with the Rebec and other instruments when he was asked to give lectures on violin making.

Ron had made up twelve sets of cello ribs from beautiful (Scottish) figured maple but not got round to finishing them. He burnt those on the bonfire, along with old invoices and other papers. There was just nowhere else to keep them! Everywhere in the house was filled with things from the two rooms. Much of the quarter sawn wood we sold to another maker at a knock down price. The lot included billets of Pernambuco for making bows. It's difficult to obtain and is the best wood for making bows but only useful to bow makers! This type of wood was first imported to make dye for the cloth making industry and someone discovered that it was good for making bows. It is difficult to find pieces of straight grained Pernambuco long enough for bows and we had several pieces, but we had to let it all go. What a bargain the man had!

The house didn't look too untidy down stairs, but upstairs was complete turmoil. We managed to keep the bedrooms we were using reasonable, but you couldn't get into some rooms!

Ron decided that some of his woodworking machines would have to go and made enquiries with second hand machine dealers. All said how depressed the market was those who expressed an interest quoted silly prices and Ron said he would rather keep them than let them go at that price, but we didn't have room to keep them! He couldn't move in his workshop, he still used it for pottering about in. April came to our rescue, she put them on eBay and they were all sold and for good prices! We wouldn't know where to start to do that ourselves!

A small builder we knew made some alterations in the two rooms upstairs. He put in a partition for a shower room off what was to become a bedroom and an extra internal door at the bottom of the stairs. A friend of Ron's, who was a plumber, put in a new separate hot and cold water system, shower, toilet and feed to the other room where a kitchen would be. One day when I was out Ron was fixing a toilet paper holder on an outside wall and hit a water pipe we didn't know was there! The pressure of water went through the open door and hit the other side of the room some eighteen foot away! Fortunately, the plumber was working not far away and was able to come and fix it for us. I didn't know water could make such a mess, it even leaked under the skirting board through the wall and into the room next door! I don't know how, but it did!

An electrician in the village rewired the flatlet completely so that it was separate from our part of the house. We put in a kitchen bar at one end of what was to become the lounge and then painted and decorated it all. It took seven weeks in all to be good enough for Andrew move into! Pretty good going I thought for a pair of oldies.

We had discussed matters with Amanda just before Christmas and she suggested that we contact an Occupational Therapist to see if they could help. I phoned 'Signposts' who put our query to the right department and they said we will have to have another assessment of needs but as it was Christmas, everything had come to a standstill. Several weeks later a 'locum' OT arrived, I didn't know there were such people, but we explained what had happened. She said we should be entitled to a disablement adaptation grant and would speak to the Council. A call from her confirmed that what we were doing would be eligible for a disability grant, but not retrospectively and they were out of money until the new financial year, which started in April. We should stop what we were doing and apply to the grant making department. Then a Council spokesman phoned and asked how far we had got with the alterations and we told them that the shower was being cemented in that very day. Too late!

Later the OT said that having spoken to the Council they still had money ear marked for Andrew at the other flat. They said that I hadn't told them that he was moving! I explained that Social Services had been told and we asked them to deal with it! If the money was still ear marked for Andrew couldn't it be transferred? She said she would ask but the answer was NO! We couldn't put off the work until April, we needed a solution to our problems now, April would be too late! We paid all the expenses from our retirement savings fund and got on with it. I couldn't see why the grant shouldn't be paid as it was already ear marked for us.

Andrew, like all of us, had worked hard for as long as he could. We had always thought that the tax and other contributions that we all pay, would mean if help was needed, it would be there. But now it seems, authority will find any excuse it can, to avoid responsibilities. If Andrew was ever offered appropriate accommodation and we couldn't see that happening, we could let the flatlet or sell up and move to a smaller house. That is what we had always thought would happen as we got older.

Council Tax on the two rooms was to be separate from the main house and we should be able to have a one band reduction in our Council Tax. This was the only concession to housing a disabled person. We put his flat on the market with a heavy heart, looked forward to being mortgage free again.

Gail from Headway returned to work and was surprised that Andrew was still with us. She thought he would have been back at home in his flat by now. We explained what had happened and that he would not be going back, he was here to stay. As his circumstances had changed she would tell her line manager and see if he was still eligible for their service! I said he was still very poorly and did need help, she would see what could be done for him.

Her help was to continue for the moment and by the time of her next appointment we were in such turmoil that she couldn't really work with Andrew at all. They talked about what had to be done to organise moving his possessions when the flat was sold. This time he was downsizing from a one bedroom flat to two rooms. I asked her if she could take Andrew to the doctors to collect his prescription as it would save me going, there was so much to do. If she could do that I would pay for the petrol. She had a small petrol allowance for that sort of job she said and would be happy to take him.

Eventually Andrew, Amanda, myself and the Social Services, who were reviewing Headway's input, all agreed that we didn't need two lots of support and Amanda's was more appropriate so Headway was withdrawn. It was understood that it might be a while before Andrew would be well enough to take control of his day to day life again. Nothing had changed much as far as his health was concerned, it was pretty awful. The sickness, diarrhoea, chronic persistent pain all contributed to his depression.

The oedema (swelling) came again and this time fortunately it coincided with an appointment with the gastroenterologist. I had never seen Andrew so enlarged before, even his eyelids were swollen, his face was fat as were his tummy, legs, ankles and even the under soles of his feet! It was difficult to find a belt to hold his trousers up, Ron in his usual fashion found a way around the problem. We used a leather bass carrying strap, designed to go round the middle of a bass to make it easier to carry. We made another hole in it with a hole punch and it did the job. Although he found it difficult to walk we got him to outpatients department.

The consultant was most concerned at his condition and thought it might be nephrotic syndrome, a kidney problem. He wanted Andrew to go into hospital at once, but Andrew said no, he didn't want to do that. I whispered to him, "Perhaps you mean can it be treated at home please?" A 24 hour urine collection was needed and we said we would collect it at home and deliver it to the laboratory, if that would be OK and it was agreed. It was good of the doctor to understand how Andrew felt about hospitals now. There was no way anyone could persuade him into hospital. The tests came back negative, it wasn't nephrotic syndrome! It was a couple of weeks before the swelling started to go down. All sorts of other tests proved negative, we know what it isn't! It was five months before all the swelling had gone.

From the PSN, a patient in America wrote.

'I don't post much but I read everything. I had my TP (total Pancreatectomy) in 1991, before they did islet cell transplants.'

I'll come back to that later.

'They also took the spleen and gall bladder. I had the pain you are describing shortly after I was discharged. At first it wasn't associated with surgery and they wouldn't give me anything for it, not knowing what was causing it. After a few days it went away on its own. It happened a second time and I suffered at home. I'm too afraid of hospitals……. Teaching doctors about TPs isn't fun… I wish you all a pain free day!'

In America a total Pancreatectomy operation can now be done with an islet transplant. It means that the insulin producing cells are gathered from the pancreas and placed in the liver where they continue to produce insulin. So the patient doesn't become an instant diabetic due to lack of insulin. In this country the NHS does not fund this operation as they want to evaluate it first! But as no operations are done, they can't evaluate them! Eventually Diabetes UK funded ten operations! Now the operation can be evaluated and we wait to see what will happen!

And in the Midlands.

'I have recently spent over five weeks in an NHS hospital (I am a staff nurse working for the NHS - although I work on a children's ward).

I was often shocked at what I saw.

ANDREW'S STORY

Even though I was unable to eat, and on a drip I saw a dietician about three times, and then little advice was offered. I usually have over-night tube feeds at home as I am limited with what I can eat, but I was just told to persevere with the tube feeds, even though they were causing pain and vomiting, as the doctor didn't think TPN was a good idea. No explanation was offered for this, and I only saw my consultant briefly on three occasions. When I saw junior doctors, because I have a long-term condition, nobody was willing to make any decisions.

As for pain relief, I am usually on fentanyl patches and lozenges, and when I need to go to hospital I usually have pethidine as well. I have had reactions to morphine, codeine and oxycodone, which are all documented in my notes; however, doctors wanted to give them to me! The registrar insisted I wouldn't be able to tolerate pethidine if I had problems with morphine and oxycodone, and wouldn't listen when I tried to explain - he actually sat and sniggered at me when I was trying to explain why I have pethidine.

I don't think I shall be going back – unless I am left with no choice!'

*   *   *

The PALS officer arranged the case meeting. In attendance were four people from the housing department, one from Shelter, the PALS officer, my doctor, Amanda, someone from Social Services!   (I thought they had closed the file, but they came anyway) CAB myself, Ron and Andrew. As Andrew was living with us now, he could re-register with our family doctor again and the first thing he did was to refer Andrew back to the Pain Clinic!

The object of the meeting was:

1. To agree the purpose of the meeting,
2. To review Andrew's needs.
3. To review our (parents/carers) needs.
4. Housing discussion.
5. Health and Social needs.
6. Other support available.
7. The way forward.

The meeting asked Andrew to briefly explain his problems. He told them about the pump, how much it cost and how much the running costs are and said he needed benefits to pay for it, as the NHS didn't fund it, his DLA should not have to be used to pay his rent. He said how much better his diabetes is with the pump and that it saved the NHS a lot of resources in hospitalisations and future complications. The illness had robbed him of his wife, his job, his home and he had been

ANDREW'S STORY

declared bankrupt. It had robbed him of his self-confidence and self-respect and he needed help.

I briefly told them that we had spent many thousands of pounds of our retirement fund to accommodate Andrew as no one else had offered to help him and we could not see him living on the streets. In my opinion Andrew was the only person in Somerset with Childhood Hereditary Pancreatitis, it is very rare and no one here seemed to understand. No one knew anything about it, how to treat it, or how it affects people.

Ron said that our life style and Andrew's were not always compatible and how upset he was to have to burn his possessions to make room for the conversion. He regretted the lack of understanding on the part of authority.

Housing people said that after extensive investigations and advice from the Health Protection Unit, advice was that Andrew was not vulnerable and he was not homeless now! The Court date for the appeal was in March, the Court could ask them to look at their decision again but not change it. Andrew disagreed. Andrew said that ideally he would want to live apart from his parents who were retired and shouldn't have to house him or have any responsibility for him.

The council representative said that since the original application, Andrew's circumstances had changed. They also said that he would have to be 'repointed'; it made him sound like a building project! He would be considered for a general needs flat, sheltered accommodation was for over sixties only. They would see what the court said about homelessness.

Andrew's housing benefit application had been classed as defective, as information had not been forthcoming from the sale of his flat. (What rubbish!) But they would look at it again.

Our doctor said he didn't understand the terminology of the letter that Dr. Peter had signed. In any case he thought Andrew was medically vulnerable. He would write a letter to the Housing Manager and copy it to Dr. Morkane saying so.

Support from Amanda was on going, she was helping with housing and benefits issues as best she could.

Social Services said that as Andrew was now living with his parents there was no need for Headway and it had been withdrawn! Not quite what I remember but never mind! Andrew said he did need support. He relies on his parents for everything at the moment, especially transport. He was told to try Community Transport.

ANDREW'S STORY

Summary

1. Harry from the Council would review benefits.
2. Doctor to write letter of support.
3. Homeless application is to be reviewed in Court
4. Review of support.
5. Re-stated that Andrew should use Community Transport.
6. Information between housing PCT and GP to be revised. (What did that mean I asked? It means that things will get better I was told!)

Exchanges between the solicitor and the housing department continued and we really thought they were not going to let this get as far as court, then suddenly their attitude changed, the co-operation stopped and they, 'were inclined to let it go to court and see what happened'!

I thought things were going to get better!

*   *   *

A few weeks later a young lady arrived with a 'trainee', to reassess Andrew's 'points'. He was tall, thickset and wore a dark suit. I thought I wouldn't like to meet you on a dark night! He took absolutely no interest in what she was saying or doing. I though to myself, they send security guards with their employees now, we must be considered dangerous!

I asked this lady if she had read the first social worker's report on Andrew and she said she had seen it. I asked again, have you read it and again she said she had seen it! Again I asked, but have you read it. Eventually she admitted she had not. I requested that she did. We never heard from her again.

Through the window when they left I saw both of them on their mobile phones, reporting back to base I guess.

        *   *   *

There was a new adviser at DIAS when I phoned. Talking things over with her she said there was a drop-in slot at the local psychiatric clinic and anyone could refer themselves! Just phone and make an appointment, they like to know if someone is going although it didn't matter if they didn't.

I made an appointment for the next day and told Andrew I was going to the clinic at Park House, he wanted to know why. I said that I just wanted to check things out and to ask if there was anything more I could do in any way. He asked if he could

ANDREW'S STORY

come and I said yes of course. We met the Community Psychiatric Nurse, it was as easy as that, just a phone call and no one had ever told me before! I introduced Andrew to her and said he wanted to come in to the interview with me. I began to tell her that no one seems to take him seriously here, how Dr. Knight was the only one who seemed prepared to help him. Soon Andrew was answering for himself. And with her careful and sensitive questioning I was able for the first time in a very long time it seemed, leave it to a professional.

She would send a report of our meeting to Andrew's GP with a copy to us and another one to the Care Co-ordinator at Park House. I had confidence that she would and she was as good as her word. Her report spoke volumes, in such a short time she had managed to grasp such a lot of the problems that no one else seemed to understand.

'Further to my fax, this is to update you regarding the above gentleman, as to the outcome of his assessment through the duty crisis slot at Park House.

He presented with his mother as a result of self-referral due to chronic pain from Pancreatitis, deep depression and diabetes. I am sure you are aware of his medical history.

Andrew stated that he had been referred to Park House in the past but was unable to attend appointments due to not being well, so his case had been closed. He did state however that he had received some input from the psychiatrist at Grove Park in the past which he had found beneficial.

He presented as in mood, speech and behaviour, but was rather quiet throughout the assessment and at one point became quite tearful. He also had to leave the room on several occasions due to his physical difficulties. (Toilet)!

He described having mood changes with a desire to 'hide away and avoid going anywhere', with no motivation, poor energy levels and an inability to gain pleasure from things.

In addition he reported having 'nothing to look forward to and having no hope for the future other than that he may die which would solve his problems'. He said he had 'contemplated suicide but felt unable to act on these thoughts due to the effects it would have on his family' He reported having these feelings since the break of his marriage and the loss of his job in 2001/2002. He also reported a disrupted sleep pattern due to his pain with him not going to bed until five or six am and then waking at 4pm.

ANDREW'S STORY

He reports feeling socially isolated and says he has no social systems other than his parents whom he is currently living with. This is a result of financial problems due to loss of his job and being unable to pay his mortgage. He says he is unable to claim housing benefit so had to move home. His mother's view is that he needs help with domestic care as he 'can't care for himself and needs a reason to get out of bed'.

Andrew felt he needed help with domestic support and in managing practical chores. He also felt he would benefit from emotional support to aid him in coping with his low mood as a result of his physical disabilities and associated life events and to come to terms with his situation. I believe he has been prescribed seroxat to aid his mood but to date it has not been found to be beneficial.

While he does receive some support through a housing association for an hour a week and some limited input from Social Services it seems they are limited in what they can do by the complexities of his difficulties.

I do think this gentleman would benefit from a full assessment of his health and social care needs as he reports not having been able to access sufficient support yet to adequately meet his needs. I would also recommend a carer's assessment be offered to his mother, which may provide additional support.

To this effect I have put a referral through to the CMHT (Community Mental Health Team) who I am sure will keep you fully informed of any future plans/ assessments outcomes.

Joy.'

Well Joy certainly knows her stuff!

One month later, I had my assessment and my husband had his some weeks after that. It was a new role for the young lady who came to see us and she was feeling her way through this new post. Later she said I should have assessed you together, next time! It seems the government in its wisdom has said that carer's needs are important and their role should be recognised and supported. I later read in a Carers UK report that carers save the Government fifty seven billion pounds a year!

It's official then, we are his carers, funny no one asked us if we were OK about it! We were told that we might be able to apply for a Carers Allowance, but after looking into it, our support worker said, as we were receiving State Pension, we didn't qualify! It was only for people in work! Can that really be true, are our needs less important because we have reached an age where we receive state pension? I made enquires of my MP, yes it's true, we are not entitled to a carers allowance because we receive state pension!

There was nothing our carer support worker could do for us. Maybe the money the assessment cost could have been better spent helping Andrew, or me! Why do adults have to rely on retired parents for help when they have worked and contributed to the system as much as they can? You think the system is there as a safety net if things go wrong, well it's not...

The day arrived for the court hearing. Our barrister was a nice young man, caring, thoughtful and I thought, good at his job. The solicitor was there and John from Shelter came to see how things were going. The Judge was not helpful to our side, picking holes in every little thing he could. He asked Andrew to take the stand, which we didn't expect and I think the Dean's barrister thought Andrew would be a push over, saying anything they tried to lead him into, but he didn't. Andrew said that he was an adult and as a medically vulnerable person, was entitled to be housed as such. He shouldn't have to rely on the charity of his ageing parents. He had worked for as long as he could, but now he couldn't work and needed help. He had lost his job, his wife, his home and was bankrupt and it wasn't his fault that he was ill; he had always done his best.

Being able to speak up for himself showed, Judge Cotterill said, that Andrew was not depressed, he showed resilience and that he could cope with life! In fact the judge said he was not medically vulnerable at all and he was getting better! (Was the judge a doctor as well?) Andrew could not properly be described as vulnerable! (The Disability Discrimination Act says he is!)

The Judge said he had been asked if it were reasonable for him (Andrew) to stay where he was. Who asked that, I don't know? Judge Cotterill said that many young people go home to their parents and although not ideal he was sure our relationship was not so fractious that we were likely to eject him from our property! What has that got to do with the case before him I asked myself.

The fact that the Office of the Deputy Prime Minister says that where a person is covered by the Disability Discrimination Act, they are medically vulnerable in housing terms was over looked. In his summing up the judge said that it was the Housing Department's role to make decisions and where advice was given, it should be relied on. The PCT said Andrew was not vulnerable, and then he was not. Case dismissed and no, we could not appeal!

The housing department were delighted and John said he could not believe what he was hearing! We sat and talked about the case in a side room at the court after it was all over. Andrew was outside smoking and John went out to be with him. The solicitor said, "That judge sits on a lot of the family courts and has a reputation of always backing authority against parents who dare to challenge authority'. The barrister said that we could go directly to the Court of Appeal and it was agreed that this is what we would do.

The appeal was prepared and started by saying that the Judge had to decide on the meaning of the word vulnerable. There were lists of examples from other cases, judgements and so on and following those, it said that the Judge had used the wrong test. Given that the whole case centred on whether or not Andrew was vulnerable the Judge's failure to use the correct test renders the decision flawed.

It went on to say that, as the appellant was claiming vulnerability due to physical disability, it was incumbent upon the respondent to take medical opinion and quoted: R. V. Lambeth LBC ex parte Carroll;

Where the applicant claims to be vulnerable for medical reasons or where, on making proper enquiries it is apparent to the authorities that such is his claim, it is both proper and necessary, as part of the enquiries which the authorities are under a duty to make, to take and consider a medical opinion, unless the applicant's condition renders him so obviously vulnerable that it is not necessary.

The Judge has said that the questions asked by the PCT were, 'singularly irrelevant' and the exercise carried out by the respondent fell far short of the standard required by ex parte Carroll. The appellant was asserting that as a result of his physical disability, he would be less able to fend for himself than an ordinary homeless person so that he would suffer injury or detriment. The respondent asked no questions about these disabilities but asked 'singularly irrelevant' questions.

The inevitable conclusion is that the Appellant was not assessed properly and the Judge was wrong to hold otherwise.

It was submitted that in purporting to delegate its decision making process, the respondent had acted unlawfully. The Judge stated that, "I find the enquiries are entirely proper and were not delegated. If the local authority does not accept the opinion of the GP then it can require an explanation but it would be imprudent not to act on an opinion provided by someone who is qualified to provide it."

The Judge was wrong to make this finding. The two questions asked were about the Appellant's mobility and mental health. The doctor was asked to simply tick a box, yes or no. It ought to have asked the GP to supply it with a list of the Appellant's complaints and their effects and their consequences, it could then decide for itself whether the combination was sufficient to render him less able to fend for himself than an ordinary homeless person so that he would suffer injury or detriment. By following the course it did, the Council did not decide for itself, it simply followed the GP's view.

It is difficult to over state the Appellants symptoms. As Dr. Knight stated in his letter to Dr. Peter, the Appellant suffers from the following:

Chronic relapsing Pancreatitis

Diabetes

Pancreatectomy and major bowel surgery

Persistent abdominal pain

Brenda Prentice

Persistently abnormal liver

Severe steatorrhoea (a severe form of diarrhoea)

Severe depression.

His clinical condition is likely to follow inexorable course of deterioration and is likely to culminate in his death.

The Judge had dismissed the appeal, stating, "It may be that another person could have reached a view more sympathetic to the Appellant but that is not enough to interfere with the decision. This is the case, even if I myself might have reached a different decision on the evidence available. This is not enough to make it an irrational decision."

The evidence before the Respondent was sufficient to render any decision that the Appellant was not vulnerable irrational. It is inconceivable that in the light of these symptoms the Appellant is no less able to fend for himself than an ordinary homeless person so that he would suffer injury or detriment in circumstances where a less vulnerable person would be able to cope without harmful effects.

It is difficult to conceive of any applicant more vulnerable as a result of his physical and mental symptoms than that of the Appellant. Indeed if

ANDREW'S STORY

applications such as the Appellant's are dismissed, it is not easy to envisage any application based on physical or mental disability succeeding.

The Appellant submits first that the Respondents decision be quashed and secondly that the court should declare that the Respondent is vulnerable as defined by Section 189(1) of the Housing Act. 1996.

The appeal was sent to the Royal Court of Justice in the Strand.
Well, that should do it!

Our application was considered by the Court of Appeal, Civil Division. Refused! The six lines of hand written words, the important ones were almost unreadable!

Rule 52.3 applies.

Rule 52.3 Decision on an application for a second appeal. The Judge will not give permission unless he or she considered that the appeal would raise an important point of principle or practice or, there is some other compelling reason for the Court of Appeal to hear it.

How about Justice as a principle, does that have anything to do with the law? I don't think it has, money buys lawyers and they interpret the law and it has nothing to do with justice! It's all a game of chance, the chance that the judge would be fair and impartial.

I phoned the Court to ask, "Who is Sir William Aldus that made this decision," I was told, "He is a retired Judge." "If he is retired why did he consider our case," I asked? "Well, he sometimes comes in to help out if we are busy!"

ANDREW'S STORY

Chapter 12

A Cry for Help?

We were woken up one night at 3am by a loud sort of bang. I always knew if Andrew couldn't sleep and was still up as his light shone on to the garden and I could see the reflection out of our window. I said he has just dropped something and turned over to go back to sleep. Ron was more concerned and went down our stairs, to go to the other end of the house to his flat. He came back saying, it's Andrew, he's on our stairs unconscious. I flew out of bed, we tried to move him but he was a dead weight, with difficulty we got him off the stairs and in a more comfortable position on the floor in the hall.

I was sure it was a diabetic black out and ran to fetch his blood test kit, but although I had watched him take his BG so many times, I had not actually done it for him and now I couldn't remember how the machine worked. We called the emergency service and they were here in twenty minutes. They also thought it could be a 'hypo' and tested his BG, it was 2.3. I've known it lower than that and he has not lost consciousness, they rubbed jell on his gums and soon he began to rouse and opened his eyes. We then gave him a sweet sugar drink and he slipped in and out of sleep, eventually waking up. His pupils were like pin picks and one of the medics said, "Has he been out tonight? Do you think he could have taken something he shouldn't?" I said that he was very ill and, no he hadn't been out. He was prescribed morphine based medication for pain and that was why his pupils were so small. "He must have had quite a dose then," he said. They asked about the illness and so we explained again what it was all about. I think I should make a recording of it!

Andrew was beginning to take an interest in what was happening around him and we told him what had happened. He remembered nothing. He said he was in great pain, had they anything for pain control on them, "No mate, we don't carry that sort of thing, asking for trouble isn't it? If you need that we can take you into hospital."
"'No," Andrew said, "It's OK," and they left after being here for half an hour. It was excellent service as ever, from the emergency team! Ten minutes later Andrew said, "Will you take me to Grove Park, I can't stand this pain any longer." So having sent the ambulance away, I took him to hospital.

In A&E we explained again what had happened, they gave him an injection of Pethidine and we went home, it was 5am.

ANDREW'S STORY

Two weeks later April was home for a long weekend. She was a bit miserable as she was going to Mexico and needed new clothes; she said, "I have a new case and nothing to put in it!" At the age of thirty five in 2003, April had decided to try to trace her birth father. She was curious to know her background and I could understand that. I think I would have been curious in her position. In this situation there are two choices, go with it, or not. If you don't, you risk losing your child. You simply have to trust there is a good enough relationship to make room for everyone. I knew her heart was big enough for all of us and made sure she understood we supported her and it would not cause us any problem. Having said that, I did have to swallow hard and hope it would all be alright in the end!

For April it was not difficult to find her birth dad, there was help from Social Services; I call it the 'find a dad office'! April's birth father was Scottish and now had a Mexican wife, two step children and a daughter! They lived on the south coast, but the older children had left home now. Interestingly, BD (birth dad) had told the family about April and they all wanted to know what took her so long to find them! BD asked her if she hated him for what had happened so long ago, she assured him that she didn't hate anyone and just wanted to get to know them. He said, "I don't have any money!" "Well that's OK," responded

April, "Neither do I!" For April it was wonderful to have the opportunity to meet them all and be able to converse with them in Spanish. She was always happy to use any language she knew at any opportunity.

She was made a welcome member of their family and they wanted to know all about her life and us. Eventually BD said he would like to meet us if we wouldn't mind, how could we say no? He made the journey to meet us here and I wonder if we were being examined to see if we came up to expectation. I shouldn't have been concerned, he was more worried at meeting us and he just wanted to say thank you, for all you have done for April. He said, we had brought her up be kind and considerate, she was talented and well educated and how grateful he was that she had been happy as a child (Was she? That's nice to know! You never can be sure.) He could never thank us enough! That was nice of him, he didn't have to say and I think it took a lot of courage on his part to meet us. We all had to try to get on for April's sake; it was her well being that we all cared most about.

BD said that April's BM (birth Mum) went back to Canada and he lost contact with her. He later phoned April to say there was a family business in Canada and he looked it up on the web. It was still there! He phoned BM and she recognised his

ANDREW'S STORY

voice straight away. She guessed why he had phoned and said she would like to meet April, but needed sometime to break the news to other members of the family. It was something she had never told them. So any contact was postponed for a while until April's other half brother and sister had been told of her existence. I didn't envy BM, how difficult to tell your children about a long ago deeply hidden secret.

It was April's two brothers, here, that took events with a little distress; I had to work hard to assure them that it didn't mean that she was rejecting us! She was just curious to know what her background was and they soon came to see that I was right. We just needed to give her a little time.

In the meantime the other family were going to Mexico to visit
In-laws and asked April to go with them, they all knew about her it seemed! BD said that as he had missed a lot of birthdays and Christmases, he would like to pay her fare…!

The long weekend started late on Thursday night when we picked April up from the station and as Andrew had an appointment with Dr. Knight the next day, we thought we would go shopping in Bristol to see if we could find anything to fill the suitcase.

I usually went with Andrew to see Dr. Knight, but he said he would go on his own and meet us afterwards in the shopping precinct. The hospital is near the shopping centre and we could have tea there. The mobile phone rang and we all met up. April hates shopping and was getting very dispirited at not finding anything she liked, or if she did, it didn't fit! Andrew on the other hand loves shopping and spending money, anyone's money! Although now he was trying to be better and more responsible at managing his money!

He and I looked at clothes that might do and I took them to April in the changing room. "How did you get on?" I asked him. "Dr. Knight said I had to tell you." "Tell me what?" "About my last blackout, it wasn't an accident. I think she would like this skirt, I'll take it to her!" When he came back I said. "Andrew, what are you trying to tell me, what wasn't an accident?" "When I collapsed on the stairs." "Did Dr. Knight know about it then?" I asked. "Yes, I think he had a report about it from Grove Park. I told him I just had a low, but he said it can't happen like that with a pump. I had to admit, I did it myself, I turned the pump up high and delivered more and more insulin. I knew it would give me a low and I hoped I wouldn't wake up." I was stunned, it never occurred to me. Andrew said, "He asked if you knew and I said no. He told me to tell you the truth; it was my first step towards healing." April called, "Can you find this

218

ANDREW'S STORY

in a bigger size?" And off he went to look.
"Andrew, can we talk about this when we get
home?" "Yes."

I tried, for April's sake, to be happy and interested
in her shopping trip, but it was hard. Andrew had
found so many things that she looked nice in, he
was in his element. The shop assistants were
amused to see him doing their job and said, "You
should be a personal shopper assistant," and he
replied, "I would like that."

At home, he went up to his flat on his own saying
he was exhausted with the trip and wanted to be
on his own. I made dinner for us all and took
some up to Andrew for later, in case he thought he
could eat it. Alone with him I asked what it was all
about and he said, "Mum, you have no idea what
it's like in the middle of the night when you can't
sleep and the pain won't go away. I just couldn't
take it any more, but I promised Dr. Knight if it
happened again I would ask for help, I won't do it
again." The tears were streaming down his face
and I felt inadequate to know what to say or how
to help him. I told him how well I thought he dealt
with his problems and I didn't think I could manage
as well as he did, I was very proud of him. In our
bedroom that night I told Ron what had happened,
but what could he say?

The next day Steve and his girlfriend came round to see April, they sat in the living room chatting when Andrew came down; he was up early for him! He then came to me in the kitchen and said, "I've told them, Dr. Knight said they must know I asked them to forgive me and said I will not do it again, I will ask for help." The poor things, what would they think, what could they say! I made a cup of tea and asked if anyone would like to go for a walk round the common?

After the weekend, it was decided that a holiday would be nice and we booked a canal boat for six weeks time. We all needed something to look forward to and to take our minds of what had happened…

Andrew later said that Dr Knight had questioned him very closely about emergency treatment when he was in our local hospital with diabetes problems. The doctor said he would write to Grove Park. Another time I overheard him say to Andrew, "I will always be here if you want to see me; next week, next month or in ten years. I'll be here waiting to see you!" Such kindness, I was overwhelmed.

This disease is such a bugger! Few seem to know anything about it let alone understand it. What could be done to bring it to the attention of people in general and some doctors! We contacted the

ANDREW'S STORY

John Peel 'Home Truths' radio programme saying that having Pancreatitis is worse than having cancer. They phoned back and Andrew and I were to be interviewed by Mr. Peel himself! We went to the local BBC studio where they contacted London and the recording took place. Andrew spoke about the disease, how it affected him and explained about his insulin pump. Then he told them how once he had turned it full on when he had been desperate and could find no respite from the pain. He didn't expect to recover from the ensuing coma.

They asked me why I thought it was worse than having cancer and I explained that the same drugs are used to treat the pain of this condition as are used for treating cancer. Generally people have a good idea what cancer is all about and have some sympathy, but with Pancreatitis there is usually no understanding and no sympathy. With cancer there was treatment and a possibility of a cure. There is no cure for this disease.

Astonishingly, there was so much feed back from listeners! Hundreds of letters were sent on to us! Some gave good advice; others suggested trying alternative treatments and some simply to express sympathy. Andrew's poignant description had touched many people. One wrote saying, I fully understand your remarks about cancer. I had cancer and was cured but it left me with another problem which is not understood and there is no understanding, no treatment, and I miss the sympathy and support I used to have.

The local paper got hold of the story and they sent a photographer. Andrew's photo was captioned with how he had tried to commit suicide by taking an overdose of insulin with his pump. Very little appeared about Pancreatitis or what it is.

*   *   *

Perhaps we could write to the Court of Appeal to explain what had happened and ask for leave to appeal again, in case we got a proper judge and not a retired substitute, and so we did. No answer, so two weeks later I wrote again. This time we had an answer, but no explanation of why I had to write twice. They simply said in answer to my question, "What have you done about my letter," they had filed it! I did explain that I would have preferred an answer, but no response from the young person on the other end of the phone.

In three weeks we had another appointment with Dr. Knight and he said he would like to see Andrew on his own. He wanted to know if Andrew had told us about what had happened and how we had reacted. Andrew was happy to tell him that we had been understanding and supportive. He told Dr. Knight that we were proud of the way he

ANDREW'S STORY

dealt with his illness and that we were sure we couldn't manage as well if it were us! Each day he got through was an achievement. We had booked a holiday and he was looking forward to that.

Dr. Knight wrote to our doctor explaining what had happened. It was such a relief for Andrew to be back with the doctor who had looked after him so well as a young man, before he left home as a student! With so many facets now to Andrew's illness, it was difficult for the doctor to grasp all that was going on at once, he needed time to adjust and get to know the situation and Andrew again.

The GP again asked for Andrew's pain management to be reviewed at the clinic, we were still waiting for an appointment. Whether as a result of what I began to call Andrew's 'hiccup', or not, I don't know, but suddenly there was an appointment with the pain psychologist, in two weeks time. I thought we had at least another six months to wait, probably longer! We still saw Rick the pins for acupuncture every few weeks.

Andrew asked me to go in to the appointment with him to see this new doctor and I told him that he should ask me to go in with him in front of her, just so that she knew it was his idea I should be there and not me pushing in where I wasn't wanted. When she came to call Andrew in to her office he stood up and turned to me saying, "Come on mum." She positioned herself between Andrew and myself and said, "No, I want to see you on your own first, we might ask your mum in later." Then turning to me she said, "We will be about fifty minutes," and lead him away.

In about twenty minutes Andrew came out and said, "Come on lets go," I said, "Which way," thinking he had come to call me in to the interview, but no, he said, "This way," and walked out of the exit. "I can't take any more of her bullshit!" He was very worked up! "What's the matter?" "I've never walked out of an appointment before, but I am now. She told me that I didn't mean to commit suicide; it was just a cry for help." I told her, "If it had been just that, I would have done it at midday where there were lots of people around, not at 3am on my own. I did mean it; I didn't expect to be found."

Oh great, just what we needed! So where was this help she thought he was crying for?

*   *   *

Our week on the Stratford and Avon Canal was wonderful, what a fantastic legacy we have been left by the navigators who built the canals and how lucky we are that enthusiastic volunteers have worked so hard to have them reopened. The weather was kind with blue, blue skies and April came for the weekend, it was August Bank Holiday. Even so it was not too crowded where we were on the canal. Sometimes it can be a bit like Clapham junction. April enjoyed the break and the peace and quiet so much that she phoned her boss and asked for a few more days off. It was great to have her company and nice to see her and her brother walking together along the canal bank enjoying each other's company, pity it wasn't for longer. Soon we came to a railway station where it was decided she would take her leave and we walked with her to the train which would take her back to London. All good things come to an end, but maybe next year....

Chapter 13

Feeling Peeved

We sold the flat and with the small profit we made, we changed our car. It was the first time we had bought a new car in many years and most probably the last new one we will have at our age! The new car has innovative technology engines, yes engines in the plural. It is an environmentally friendly hybrid car with an electric engine as well as a petrol one. Everyone asks me, "Do you plug it in?" The answer is, no, it recharges its own electric battery while the petrol engine is running. It has a little screen a bit like a TV screen which tells you if the battery is charging or discharging power which will assist the petrol engine, or using electric engine on it's own. It says how many miles per gallon it is doing and when running on electric engine alone it says 99.9 per gallon! Stamp your foot down hard and it will fall to seven MPG, ouch, that makes you think! The next screen tells the average MPG over the last five miles. The hand book say's it can do 67MPG, I have done sixty! I wonder why we still use MPG when we buy petrol in litres now. I thought the car was great, always quiet and a beautiful smooth ride. (Good for someone with pancreatic back pain who feels every pothole in the road!)

ANDREW'S STORY

I went back to the garage showroom to order new foot mats and to arrange for parking sensors to be fitted after my first little prang! The wall along our drive jumped out and just caught the bumper, or what passes for a bumper these days. The whole showroom had been restyled. No little refurbishment this, it was total commitment! I asked to see the salesman who I found to be exceptionally good at his job. He came down from upstairs and I asked him how he liked the rebuild. "Very nice," he said, "But I would prefer my desk down stairs so I can see what's going on in the showroom." I asked, "Why aren't you down stairs?" "Well," he said, "All our showrooms, throughout the whole country are standardised now, they are all the same. We have a hostess who will meet and greet customers, make coffee for them, find out what they came in for and maybe call a salesman down!" A hostess in a garage? I asked if this could be a new career move for me, was there a job going but he said they had appointed all the hostesses now! We laughed at the thought of an elderly retired woman like me being a hostess! "Couldn't you take your desk down stairs to the showroom when it's all finished?" I asked. "No, they send the policy police round to do spot checks!" We laughed again but he was plainly unhappy with the new set up.

*   *   *

At the beginning of September, just eighteen months after a review of his management had been asked for, there was an appointment at the Pain Clinic and at Andrew's request I went with him! Rick the pins was there and we talked about how he thought the treatment was going. As the pain had a long history and was deep seated Rick said it would take sometime to get to grips with. Andrew was asked if he thought it was helpful and he said it was.

Instead of the usual doctor we saw the big white chief! He said although he didn't usually see Andrew he had spent a long time with the other doctor reviewing Andrew's case. He began to conduct the appointment in a rather hostile way I thought. He told Andrew that there would be no more increases of medication he would just have to learn to live with his pain; there was nothing more that could be done for him. Andrew said that everyone knew that you get used to morphine and eventually needed more for the same effect. He knew people who were on double the dose he was prescribed. Andrew was told that he would become 'hypersensitive' if they prescribed more medication. As the doctor got more forceful Andrew became very quiet, eventually Andrew looked at me and said, "I think I like my idea better." The doctor homed in on this remark and asked what he meant. Andrew said, "I can't go on

ANDREW'S STORY

like this," and the doctor asked if he was going to try to commit suicide again. Andrew said nothing and looked at me; the doctor went on and on. "Are you intending to try again today? I will need you to see a psychiatrist now if you are." In order to try and break the tension, which in my view, had deliberately been built up, I intervened, "He can't do that today; we are going out to lunch with friends."

The doctor calmed down and then said "There is nothing more I can do for you, no more operations, injections or medications. I am discharging you from the department. The only thing I might offer you is a couple of sessions on how to manage your pain better by a change of lifestyle. But you have to accept first that nothing more can be done for you. I will write to you and you must write back to me." We got up and left.

Rick the pins ran after us and put his hand on Andrew's shoulder, "We have an appointment in two weeks, you will come to it won't you?" Andrew was too upset to answer but I said we would let him know.

Outside in the fresh air Andrew said to me, "You know what he was hankering for don't you, he wanted to section me. He just wants me off his list so it looks as through he is doing better and reducing his waiting list!" That had never occurred to me. (Section, as in the mental health act where a patient can be detained by force for their or the public's good)

Andrew kept the appointment with Rick.

At home I contacted a PSN member in Plymouth, I knew that he was using a morphine pump for pain control and I asked him how he was getting on with it. He said it was a vast improvement as the morphine could be directed on to the spot where the pain was coming from. By using it he had been able to cut right down on the amount of morphine he was taking by mouth! He gave me the name and address of the doctor (Professor) looking after him and said, "Contact him; I'm sure he will not mind."

I logged on to the Internet for information on morphine pumps and found they are made by the same company which made the insulin pump. That makes sense I suppose!

I wrote to the Professor in Plymouth and said I hoped it was OK to contact him; it was at the suggestion of one of his patients. I outlined Andrew's problems and asked if he thought it would be worth coming to see him….

By the end of September there was a case conference with the Mental Health team, attended

ANDREW'S STORY

by about seven people. I'm not sure who they all were but I thought, oh good, something might actually happen this time. Certainly the Mental Health team took Andrew more seriously than some. We went through his 'complex difficulties'; again. Andrew stated he felt that Grove Park did not offer adequate treatment or support in addressing problems of diabetic control and with managing physical pain.

It was agreed that through Park House, Andrew could be referred to the Bristol Pain Clinic! That's a step in the right direction! The local Diabetic Department were to be contacted and asked if they will treat Andrew if there were any diabetic emergencies. A one line letter came back saying they would, I hope we never have to put that to the test!

Amanda was at the case conference, still being funded to help support Andrew on tenancy, budgeting and finance issues. The Occupational Therapist will arrange a visit to see if we can have an extra hand rail on the stairs, that would save Ron a job, he had meant to do it but hadn't got round to it. Time someone else did something for a change instead of leaving it all to us!

Social Services said they would continue to support Andrew's housing application and I was dumfounded! I said they had never done that in the past why had they changed their mind. I was told they had always supported Andrew's application and I said they hadn't! Three times she insisted they had! I just gave up and the meeting moved on.

Andrew would like to continue with the Expert Patient Programme and become a tutor. It's the only (voluntary) job where the first requirement is to be chronically sick! The Expert Patient is a government initiative where chronically sick people are put on a 'training course' for six weeks. This is to help them take control of managing their condition themselves. The problem is that if some doctors think you are taking too much interest in your own care, they see this as a challenge to them and they don't like it. Fortunately, some are enlightened and welcome this. Andrew was to be put on the list to train to be an Expert Patient Tutor. He was never invited to training; I don't think the programme got of the ground, I don't know why.

Andrew was to be put on the waiting list to see one of the 'team' for counselling.

On the 'care plan', staff were told that 'Andrew often gave an appearance of coping but isolation and low mood often concealed the real truth'. The 'care co-ordinator' said of Grove Park, "There certainly are some strange dimensions going on here." There would be a review in three months.

They did recognise that Andrew was socially isolated and needed help to integrate. Gosh, are we making progress……

*   *   *

.A letter came from the Pain Clinic at Grove Park for Andrew.

'Given that you will remember that I said to you that we have now come absolutely to the end of what medicine can do for you with regard to changing your pain. There are no further injections or operations that will be of benefit. Likewise, if we continue to increase your dose of strong pain medication it is very likely that your pain will become worse in quite a short time and inevitably that quite soon you would reach a state of so-called hyper-analgesia where you get total body pain and are unable to move or function because of it.

After you had left the clinic today your mother telephoned to ask at what level of strong medication hyper-analgesia occurs, and it is impossible to say. What is possible for me to predict however, with 100% certainty, is that as we escalate the dose of your medication your pain will start to run away from us much more quickly than it has up until now.

Indeed, in the pain clinic we are much more expert at helping people to cope and manage their pain and live more meaningful lives, given the fact that they have pain.

Pending your thoughts, which we would like to hear by letter, we have not made you a further appointment to come back to our clinic.
We hope that you find this helpful for you in coming to a decision.
With very best wishes.'

A letter from the Plymouth hospital in answer to mine said,

'I have taken the liberty of speaking with Grove Park and it is my understanding that they feel they have not fully worked through all the management pathways and that they are going to call a case conference of all clinicians who have been intimately concerned with his care. In view of this it would not be appropriate to initiate further treatment at present.'

Well, you learn something every day, another case conference and I thought they were not going to make another appointment

ANDREW'S STORY

With great effort and concentration Andrew answered the letter from Grove Park, the three pages took him throughout the night to write, but he did it! First he reviewed his illness from where he came from and then said:

'Although terrified, I eventually had surgery, as much as anything to please my wife. For a few months I was pain free and able to come off methadone on my own without help. But the pain came back. We now know the operation has a 50% chance of failure. One doctor said to me, "What do you mean, you are in pain, you can't be, you've had the operation." Another time I was told I was a waste of NHS resources. In fact the experience of have Pancreatitis is very demoralizing and that is well documented! No one ever told me I would be disabled, we had to work that out for ourselves. I now take someone with me to appointments for moral support. You have told me about hyper- analgesia, I would risk that to have the edge taken off my pain.

I believe that ownership of my disease should be taken by an experienced specialist in this disease, instead of being passed around as nobody knows what to do with me. When we ask for a second opinion, we are told the doctors here are as good as any elsewhere. That may be true but I have been on their books for a very long time and a fresh pair of unbiased eyes might have something positive to add. Now just the thought of seeing another doctor makes my tummy knot up and a feeling of anxiety increases the longer I have to sit and wait.

You asked me 'where do I want to be,' I want to be a valued member of society again and not dependent on my parents. Until this excruciating all consuming pain, which women who suffer say is like having a baby without analgesia, everyday, is managed so that I can function, I do not think it will happen. I am weak, weary and tired of coping; I need help, not being treated like a drug addict.

Someone else that I know with this problem reported this from his pain specialist.

'Addiction in the sense it is usually used in, means a psychological dependence on drugs. Where it is taken to relieve chronic pain any dependency is likely to be physical, not psychological'.

I will willingly work with you if you can help me, but please don't blame me for what I can't help and you can't cure. Please work with me to make my last few years tolerable if not pain free, I know what my prognosis is, I'm not stupid.'

He then listed five different procedures either used on other sufferers or what he had read about.

Within two weeks an answer.

ANDREW'S STORY

'It is difficult to live with persistent pain and we know many people who come to our clinic find themselves looking for any treatment which might possibly be of benefit.

Firstly, it is important that you know your condition is due to the way the nerves in your body are transmitting and amplifying pain messages. That's all the nerves not just the ones near your spine or where your pancreas was. What this means is that all the specific treatment options you outline are doomed to failure. Unfortunately, these will simply not work for your condition. If we felt there was any operation or an injection that would help, we would have referred you well before now.'

Three weeks later Andrew wrote.

'I have thought long and hard about what you have said, I understand what you are saying but I hope you appreciate that for someone in my situation living every day in constant pain I have to explore any avenue and every possible treatment.

You have said that adjustment of morphine is not an option but you think you can help me live a more reasonable quality of life. I am prepared to try anything that you suggest as at the moment my life is miserable and hardly worth living. So I will take up your offer of further sessions to see if it makes any difference.

Thank you for your time and understanding and I look forward to the appointments and just pray that you are right.'

We waited for an appointment but nothing came.

*   *   *

The hospital makes a change of £10 for you to be allowed to look at your own personal file and an administrator must sit with you as it is read. Before this can happen, all third parties are asked if they have any objection to you seeing the file! Andrew's file was vast and split into four bundles. When we previously looked at them, the administrator could only spend an hour with us and we made an appointment to go back, in the event, Andrew wasn't well enough to go. Later we asked to look at Andrew's notes again and after much prevarication and a request for another £10, which I refused to pay, they sent a copy of all the notes added to the file, since we looked at them the last time.

One letter was from the pain doctor to our GP saying,

ANDREW'S STORY

'Andrew talked rather blithely about suicide but it was rather more suicidal ideation than intent. I did ask him if he had a clear intent to commit suicide before his next appointment with his psychiatrist and his mother interjected that,'He couldn't do it today because we are going out to lunch'. I think this gives us some idea of the sort of complex situation with which we are dealing.

I have written this letter today to you and I wonder what you think. We have now a very clear view, with a lot of supporting evidence, that patients can only clearly start to move forward in their lives once medicine has been put to one side and in Andrew's case medication has absolutely nothing to offer....' I see.

And another letter from the same source.

'I note that you have taken over the care of Andrew. At present his opiate usage is stabilised and his pain behaviour has been moderated over the past few years.'

And from the pain clinic doctor in Bristol who was on first name terms with the Grove Park doctor.

'This patient has been referred by the consultant psychiatrist, as you can see from his letter the

patient seems to have lost confidence with the help he was offered at Grove Park. Please send copies of any letters as it would obviously be helpful for me to know what approaches have been taken in the past.'

I turned to the Internet for help.

It became clear that the world's foremost authority on pain was Professor Patrick Wall. Before his death he transformed the understanding of pain.

From his book, 'Defeating Pain, The War on the Silent Epidemic'.

'There is a common problem which affects everyone who is in pain for long periods. This problem concerns the meaning of the word 'acceptance'. It is one thing to accept that no one has a complete solution to a particular pain condition. It is quite another to accept that nothing can be done. To demand that patients should accept the uselessness of all help is to condemn him to a feeling of betrayal, alienation and depression. The result is a downward spiral, which becomes increasingly difficult to interrupt. The hospice movement teaches us a splendid example by asserting and proving that comfort and dignity can be achieved even for those whose life is ending.

ANDREW'S STORY

To issue a command, 'to pull yourself together' to a deeply depressed, inactive patient, is an obscenity. The condition of such patients is predictable and preventable, since they were plunged into it by a sequence of dismissal and neglect. They can only be rescued by great imaginative effort as well as professional help.'

And from another of his books, 'Pain, The Science of Suffering'.

'The abandoned patient whose pain continues but in whom no damaged tissue can be detected is in serious trouble. The doctor may say, 'There is nothing wrong with you. It is all in your head'. The patient is forced to consider that he is the cause of his own suffering and is completely puzzled. If the word spreads to friends, relatives, union organizers, employer and social security officers, his loneliness is extreme. If the doctor's message is spread to others as 'Don't encourage him. It will only make it worse', the patient exists in a near vacuum.

In any Western country, there are considerable numbers of people who identify the major problem of their society as being a huge mass of swindles and manipulators who are deliberately stealing money from social services to live in luxury and do no work. The patient is now assigned to this pariah status.

People in pain have difficulty coping. Pain monopolises their world. Anger, fear, rejection and isolation clearly make matters worse. The patients conflicting sense of shame and dependency adds to their problems. When these have been deliberately triggered by the authority of doctors, the patient is in deep trouble. Very rarely, individuals can diagnose the social situation, stop complaining to others and put on an act that signals to others that they are not in pain despite their continued problems. These rare individuals may appear admirable but their public performance is a sham. For the rest of us in pain, we need comfort, support, recognition and help if we are to make the best of our days in pain. To achieve that effort, we certainly do not need a group of doctors to wash their hands of us and dump the problem entirely on our shoulders.'

We waited for an appointment from the pain clinic in Bristol but nothing came.

Another Christmas came and went with no appointments from anyone apart from Dr. Knight, the only one who seems to care or make any effort! Don't they understand urgency?

In the meantime Andrew had been using my computer and I found this email on it from him to a

ANDREW'S STORY

PSN friend. I must ask Steve to make Andrew a computer of his own!

'Just a quick note to see how things have been since Christmas and the New Year. I've been pretty ill since we last spoke and this seems to have a knock on effect on everything else! I don't know about you but I seem to be stuck in an ever decreasing downward spiral. I suffer from very bad pain and vomiting all the time and because of this I don't have the confidence to leave the house just in case I am sick. And because I don't leave the house, I get bored and depressed which gives me more time to think about the pain, which seems to get worse and so I get more depressed! I can't seem to break the cycle and no one seems to be able to help despite writing letters to my local hospital where I am supposed to be under the care of my pain management consultant, he has basically said that he does not know what to do and yet he is not willing to refer me to other pain management consultants that could possibly help.

Whatever I do to try and help myself, or find other experts that could possibly help, I run up against brick walls or obstacles! I really feel like I have come to the end of the road and think I have only one option left. The doctors and consultants have run out of options and they say it's up to me now to manage my pain, but I can't. I have thought through all the options and there seems to be only one sensible thing left to do. I have tried this before but was not successful. The only thing that has stopped me so far is the effect that it would have on my mum, dad, brother and sister. I don't want to hurt them but I don't know how much longer I can put up with the pain. Only I can make this decision and maybe in the long run my family would understand and maybe forgive me, I don't know.

Do you ever get this down and depressed? Do you feel like you have got to the end of your tether? Or maybe the pain isn't so bad in your case?

It is getting late now and the pain is always worse as I get more tired so I will have to sign off now and go to bed and hope that I can sleep, it seems that it is the only time I get a break from the pain nowadays. I must go now and I apologise for going on but it helps to talk to some one who understands what this illness is like. I hope that things are better at your end and I look forward to hearing from you soon.

Andrew'

And an answer.

'I'm sorry to hear things are no better for you and yes I understand completely, I've spent the last

ANDREW'S STORY

seven years in exactly the same cycle but three months ago I got totally to the end of my tether, much like yourself. I felt the only option left to be a final one. Before I took this option and feeling I had nothing left to lose I re-approached my pain team which were equally as unhelpful as yours and demanded they put me on a course of medication I had prior to my operation. The only one I ever had which was strong enough to kill the pain, so I know they work. They don't want to give it to me as they are opiates and addictive but I don't care about that; I just want to be pain free. As far as I was concerned I saw it as obvious if I were to gain any life at all.

I demanded they helped me and put me back on slow release morphine and gave me break through pain killer tablets. I got laxatives, as you know they do bung you up which also causes pain, and for sickness, I got metroclopamide. It has totally transformed my life and I got about 70% function back which was a vast improvement but I wasn't satisfied and after three months I eventually went back to my GP and explained that I still had pain although not as bad as before and without hesitation he doubled it! Since then I can function as a normal human being for 95% of the time and it is fantastic!

I am living instead of existing in agony twenty four hours a day such as you are now, and I'm moving house. I contacted Social Services and they have given me an advocate, she has organised for me to go to a day centre for people with chronic pain, I go twice a week and they organise transport, it's fantastic to be in the company of people who understand just what constant pain is like!

I really would like you to go down the same path as myself and demand and shout until you get the medication that will turn your life round totally and give you a reason to live. I am really worried that you are about to do something drastic that could be avoided if you try this avenue first. If no joy then demand that your GP refer you elsewhere to someone that can help as opposed to hinder and just keep fobbing you off. You have absolutely nothing left to lose.

I know it's hard, I've wanted to end it all so many times and the only thing that has stopped me is the thought of my seven year old daughter growing up without a Dad.

I would feel a whole lot better if you told me you would do this, you are not out there to makes friends with these people, they get paid a great deal of money to help people like us.'

While we were waiting for the appointment from Bristol for the pain clinic and after a letter from Andrew begging for a higher dose of pain killer,

ANDREW'S STORY

our GP let the dose rise, a lot! He was beginning to understand the problems, although he didn't really approve of increasing it by so much. True enough though; Andrew was able to function better with the higher dose. The stairs were not such a problem, he came down to socialise with us and have a cup of tea. He started coming out with us to doing his own shopping again and on the odd occasion coming out with us to socialise. While the pain hadn't gone, he was able to live with it a little better, it wasn't quite so paralysing. The depression did not change.

We heard nothing of the case conference to be organised by the pain department and three months later I wrote to them asking if it could be expedited as Andrew was far from well. I also asked what operations he meant when he said; there will be no more operations, injections etc. I couldn't remember any. I received an answer saying it wasn't easy to find a date to suit everyone. I then saw a copy of a letter from the pain clinic to other clinicians saying,

'They have self-referred to Plymouth and the psychiatrist has referred them to Bristol pain clinic. The gastroenterologist has referred him to a London hospital.'

The gastroenterologist then sent a letter to all those concerned saying he hadn't referred Andrew anywhere, and eventually it all fizzled out, I feel there was no real intent. No need to wait for them any longer! The fact that Andrew was still in intense pain didn't seem to enter their equation…

Eventually, in April 2006 a letter from the pain clinic to Andrew and myself ending with, you have now been formally discharged from the pain clinic and I cannot enter into further correspondence regarding your case.

From the PSN. An American view point.

'Thanks for your prayers. Prayer has pulled us through for three years now. I just got home from seeing my husband at the hospital. They always have a hard time controlling his pain but once they finally get that settled he's OK. He always requires more medication than any nurse is ever used to giving. The amounts he can tolerate would usually make someone stop breathing; it just makes him able to tolerate the pain. Is this a common problem with Pancreatitis? It seems like they always think he is just wanting drugs and over reacting.'

In order to try and get on top of the sickness and steatorrhoea the gastroenterologist was arranging for Andrew to have investigations as an in-patient in Grove Park, but decided to wait until after the

ANDREW'S STORY

'case conference'. With that option gone the
doctor made arrangements to admit Andrew

Andrew was not very happy about going into
hospital again but the doctor said he would make
the stay as short as possible and Andrew
eventually agreed. Weeks went by with beds
being available and then at the last minute being
taken by 'emergency patients'. Each time Andrew
got more worked up about going to hospital, as he
said, "I've been in so many times with no result,
why should this time be different?" Eventually
there was a bed on Thursday and I took a
reluctant patient to the ward at 4pm. The
Consultant was on the ward, he came over shook
hands and said it was nice to see him; he would
leave his team to settle him in. The junior doctor
said, "We can't find your notes, they have been
sent for but they haven't arrived yet." I told her
that the notes were not stored in the hospital but in
another building twenty minutes drive away. She
said she had only started at the hospital yesterday
and didn't know where they were kept.

The next day the notes came and the doctor said,
"It doesn't say why you are here and we are not
sure what tests to run." Andrew told them that he
thought they were to weigh everything that he
passed or vomited. A form was brought with
crude hand drawn pictures as to what shape
stools were passed and Andrew was to tick the

nearest likeness! I arrived to visit that evening and was told that nothing much was happening. Andrew said the consultant wouldn't be round until Monday at the earliest and as the junior doctors didn't really know what was going on; couldn't he go home for the weekend? We asked the sister; "No," she said, "If you go you will find someone else in your bed when you get back." "What happens?" I asked, thinking about the policy police at the garage, "Do the bed police come round and check up!" I did have a smile on my face and my tongue in my cheek but she was not amused!

"I have to fill in a form each day at 8pm to say how many beds are not occupied." Eventually Andrew was allowed to go home for the day and he had to be back at 8pm each night to sit on his bed! He was not happy at the attitude, as usual.

As I was in the hospital I thought I would visit someone I knew from my walking club, she was there to have tests for suspected bone cancer. In her ward I was asked by one of the staff if they could help and I said I couldn't see Sue, which bed was she in? "Oh you missed her by about half an hour; she has gone home for the weekend, back on Monday!" No wonder Andrew feels peeved.

ANDREW'S STORY

On Monday the consultant did a ward round. He told his team that although Andrew looked very well, he in fact was very sick and had been for a long time. They should learn from this and not assume that if someone looks well that they are it's not always the case, as with Andrew.

On Monday, there was no steatorrhoea! We couldn't remember the last time he had a day free of it. Knowing looks from the staff! On Tuesday the bedpan was left in the toilet with paper over it and the nurse informed he was so embarrassed at all this. The nurse should have taken it down to the laboratory but she was busy. The next time he used the bedpan, the first was still there smelling awful! But by the next time both bowls were gone, he assumed to the lab. But the young doctor asked him what he had done with them. He didn't know where they were, hadn't the nurse taken them? And no, he hadn't flushed them away. Of course he hadn't, why should he? The nurse said they weren't there when she went to collect them and take them to the lab. Maybe the cleaners had been cleaning! There followed quite a few words with the staff and Andrew. When I arrived to visit he said, "Take me home, I've had enough of this!" He had been there five days with nothing to show for it other than bad feeling all around.

He wrote to the consultant saying that, "We have both been let down by the young doctor and the staff." I wrote apologising for all the problems, couldn't I collect what was needed at home and deliver it on a twice daily basis to the lab. I was so grateful that Andrew wasn't discharged from the care of this specialist and that he was more understanding than I thought he would be, thank goodness. It was agreed that they would look for suitable containers and we would do the collection at home. The Gastro doctor was beginning to understand Andrew and work with him, such a relief. Not like some departments!

This doctor's mind runs at the speed of an express train, it's so interesting to observe, but my mind struggles to be a freight train and keeping up with him is a challenge! In fact I sometimes wonder if mine has come to the buffers!

I didn't hear from the hospital for several weeks and when I phoned the secretary she said, "So far we can't get the right containers." I said I would pop down to Lakeland and buy some, just let me know what size to get! Later I was told, "They don't have the containers as they don't do that test in the lab any more," oh dear, what now! We managed to retain a good relationship with the consultant, I was very grateful for that and he said he would think again!

*   *   *

ANDREW'S STORY

Eight months later and with the blessing of the mental health team, I was to write to Bristol pain clinic and asked why we hadn't had an appointment. At the same time I had a long chat with our GP who was feeling uncomfortable prescribing such huge doses of pain medication. As he said, "Post Shipman, everyone is walking on egg shells!" He eventually referred us to St. Thomas's in London. There had been a series of morning TV programmes from there which a friend had seen. She video taped one of the programmes, which was on pain management and gave it to me, it was very impressive and we thought it was worth asking them if they could see Andrew.

I got in contact with the consultant and asked if he could see us privately and within a week we had an appointment. After the years of waiting for something to happen in Somerset, that was amazing! The GP faxed a referral and in a few days we went to London to see the consultant.

He was a real gentleman in the old fashion sense, with a quiet authority about him. I would have guessed he was east European. He asked if Andrew was working and was told, "No, I was sacked and I can't work any more." The consultant's conclusion was that, "You are too young to be given up on, I can't promise to find a cure, but I can promise to try!" That's all we ever asked! "I will see you as an NHS patient as treatment can become very expensive and you should be treated by the NHS, it's your right." I could have cried!

I had written to Bristol asking why we had not received an appointment. They said they were sorry, the appointment had been left on the pending list and it wasn't until I had written they realised there had been an oversight. They said they had written to Grove Park and there hadn't been a reply, they had faxed a request for information that day. They apologised but understood that we now had an appointment at St. Thomas's and no longer needed an appointment at Bristol. I left it at that.

Two months later we received a questionnaire prior to an appointment to be made to attend Bristol Pain clinic! Andrew was very upset, "What is going on?" He asked. "I thought that was behind us now." I wrote back saying that I take it that a response had been received from Grove Park and we would like to see it. Needless to say, we were not privy to that information, simply being told to ask Grove Park for it.

Thinking along these lines and our fruitless trip to Liverpool, I wrote to that hospital asking to see the referral letter from Dr. Peter. My letter was ignored, so I wrote again. Still nothing and as I had to speak to the solicitor, I asked him to write on our behalf. He said we were entitled to see the referral and didn't need to pay him to write a letter, but I said we wanted it over and done with and not for it to drag on. "While you are writing, ask for the whole file please," I said as an after thought!

He wrote and within seven days we had the whole file and an apology for the delay! I wrote back and said if they were sorry would they like to contribute to the solicitor's bill but there was no answer.

From the PSN

'If, like me you are unfortunate enough to misplace your pancreas I am afraid the chances of being free of pain is very small indeed. (His pancreas had completely consumed itself) *All sufferers I know that are surviving without a pancreas still have pain and frequent attacks. Level 8-10 pain attacks are rarer though. I know of one who has survived without a pancreas but his pain levels are so high that he lives on morphine 24/7.'*

The referral letter to Liverpool from Dr. Peter said:

2nd July 2003.

'I gather you are going to see this thirty two year old man next week. He has had a partial

Pancreatectomy and a Whipple's procedure and now has an insulin pump. I will extract some correspondence, copy them and forward them by mail.'

(Actually, it was a total Pancreatectomy, didn't he know that)?

3rd. July 2003

'Thank you for seeing this gentleman with chronic Pancreatitis whose main symptoms are of chronic pain, mal-absorption and diabetes. He is usually looking fit and well when he presents himself in public, but I suspect he goes home and feels sorry for himself, in pain and then over-uses his medication. Consequently, many of his consultations are for extra opiates and not very satisfactory to either side. I am grateful for your expert advice.'

His letter definitely stated 'with chronic Pancreatitis'! I had often been corrected by medics if I said, he has Pancreatitis. I would be told he couldn't have Pancreatitis as he didn't have a pancreas. Did Dr. Peter know, I wondered if Andrew had a pancreas, a partial pancreas, or no pancreas at all?

ANDREW'S STORY

There was a letter from the doctor in Liverpool to the GP after our appointment, three pages long, we had never been sent a copy of it or been told about. We didn't know it existed! The interesting points were,

'Andrew had started drinking age twenty nine and drinks no more than two units a week and has continued this habit. He smokes thirty cigarettes a day which he has been doing for the last nineteen years.'

(Having tried alcohol after his total Pancreatectomy, he didn't like it and asked how anyone could drink that stuff for pleasure! He remains what he had always been, teetotal. I think I would have noticed if he smoked thirty a day aged ten! I hope this man is more accurate in other matters.)

'On 18th June 1997 he underwent a left Pancreatectomy in Exeter Hospital, (only ten years out, it was 1987, never mind*!) He subsequently underwent a completion total Pancreatectomy on 26th February1999.* (Two years later! No*) Following this he had no pain for nine months but subsequently started sensing pancreatic pain and has since steadily increased his analgesia. He describes his condition as severely restricted.*

He opens his bowls three times a day with some steatorrhoea and takes 225,000 units of Creon per day.

He had an appendicectomy at the age of fifteen years old! His father is a violin maker, (what does that have to do with anything)?

The presentation and history was fairly typical. What was disappointing however, was his continued opioid dependency.
It should be possible to phase out opiate use and return to a normal existence. I mentioned to him the possibility of bilateral thoracoscopic sympathectomy. This should provide instant pain relief but unless he was determined to stay off opiates and give a strong practical demonstration of this preoperatively then this procedure should not be undertaken on him. (I just don't understand that, why?)

He has had a splenectomy and it was not clear that he had been vaccinated against haemophilus and pneumococcus. He should also take regular oral Penicillin.'

(He definitely does have a spleen, so he doesn't need the vaccination, but why didn't Dr. Peter ask about this!)

He also wrote about Genetics and Nutrition.

ANDREW'S STORY

Then, on steatorrhoea again,

'His intake of Creon is on the low side. On average these patients require of the order of 100,000 to 800,000 lipid units per day. Therefore, I would recommend that he switch to Creon 40,000 capsules and has ten to twelve of these a day.'

(Actually the dose must be based on the amount of fat in food eaten, if more creon is taken than needed it does not 'switch off', it goes on digesting what ever it comes into contact with. Andrew was told by a nutritionist if his bottom was sore to cut down on creon at once until it was better, it could be the creon digesting his backside).

And finally,

'The response by Andrew to the above was one of disappointment. He was disappointed that there was no magic formula for him and resented the idea that there was no magic formula for his pain problem.'

It wasn't magic we wanted. It seems there was an operation which could have been tried after all.

I had heard through the PSN that this doctor didn't like patients to be on morphine at all, especially if they had had a total Pancreatectomy. It was his own team's research that said there was a 50% success rate with this operation where it had been performed for reasons of pain. So why was he so concerned that some people still needed morphine when the operation failed? I don't understand. It is a proven fact of their own department that for some, this operation has no benefit at all; they are worse off after it, than before.

Looking at the file letters Dr. Peter had sent to Liverpool, one was dated 1991 when Andrew was just twenty. It was from Grove Park to a hospital in Plymouth where he had been a student some fifteen years ago. It said,

'Yes, we know Andrew well and although I don't have his notes in front of me his Pancreatitis is alcohol induced and he abuses his analgesia'.

Further on it said that

'The family relationship is strained and he does not get on with his father'.

I was stunned. How could any doctor write such a letter?

The notes about the operation in 1999 which I had sent to Liverpool also came back. They had cost me £17 to have copied at Grove Park! Looking at

ANDREW'S STORY

them again I still found the hand writing difficult to understand as before, but with time I deciphered some of them. It seems the pancreas was not the only thing taken out; part of the stomach, small bowl and intestine also went. Interestingly, the diabetes was difficult to control even before he was discharged, and the pain referred to as chronic. They wanted Andrew to be off all opiates before leaving hospital. I felt that was a bit unrealistic as he had been on them for sometime and it would take time to adjust to that. No appointment at any drugs rehabilitation clinic was suggested.

There were other letters from various doctors included one from Dr. Knight, thank goodness for him, we could rely on him to get it right! Altogether, it was an interesting read, but I shouldn't have had to employ a solicitor to get the notes it is our right to see them.

Now what is to be done about this letter dating from 1991, why on earth did Dr. Peter send it to Liverpool, come to that, why was it written in the first place….. It needed thinking about.

At our next meeting with Dr. Knight he again asked if Andrew was being seen by the mental health team in Taunton and again we had to say we are waiting for an appointment. This time he said I think it would be good to see someone here at our hospital and within a very short time an appointment arrived through the post! Unfortunately, it was at 9.15am. That meant getting up at 6.30am taking into account the stops needed at service stations for steatorrhoea and I asked if the appointment could be made later. In order to fit in with ward rounds and so on, it was the only time outpatients could be seen. All was not lost; I had a friend who lived in Bristol. "If we bring our sleeping bags can we stay the night?" "Yes but you don't need to bring your sleeping bags," but we took them anyway as it saved a lot of washing for one night and anyway we needed our B&B on a regular basis!

To start with Andrew wanted me to go to the appointment with him; his self confidence was very low. Each time we met, the doctor said, "You shouldn't have to come all this way, this service should be available to you in Taunton." As the meetings went on it was clear that Andrew wanted me with him and sometimes Ron came too. We covered Andrew's background, childhood, adoption, his place in the family, in fact everything that was or had been important in his life.

Over the nine sessions we had with the doctor he went into the complex health issues that spanned over twenty years. How Andrew lived in a state of constant pain and how sometimes stress can play a part in this. So he was thinking about Andrew's problems in the context of both mind and body together. Andrew admitted he was bullied at school, something we didn't know about, is this why he wants us there, so at last he can tell us things we didn't know? We talked about the number of clinicians Andrew had seen over the years and how often his needs had been overlooked and he felt he was not trusted. It appeared at times that he was not given the care he needed and it caused tension with clinicians. How he felt he received most help from outside our local authority area and that at times it felt like he was blamed for their failure. Andrew talked about how he built up a wall round him to try and protect himself from the hopelessness of it all. He tried not to show his emotion and felt he was hurting his parents if he did, when they tried so hard to help but were not able to. "We have kept in close contact with your care coordinator on the understanding that when our work is finished here you will be offered continuous psychological support from this team."

The report was sent to Andrew's current doctors and he asked that it also be sent to three consultants at Grove Park that he didn't see anymore.

*   *   *

We waited and eventually an appointment came to see a psychologist at Park House. Very nervously Andrew asked me to accompany him to the first session. I was told by the young lady that she did see young adult men without their mum's! That put me in my place, after all the co-operation we had had in Bristol, we were back to patient confidentiality, great words for hiding behind! She couldn't or wouldn't see that I also had a need to see that his treatment was right for him. As Dr. Knight had said, "You won't jell with everyone and it is important to get the right person for you." I had a part to play in seeing that people didn't get hold of the wrong end of the stick. If Andrew told half the story as he sometimes did, he would leave it to me to continue. Sometimes he found it so painful that he couldn't go on and was grateful for me to fill in the gaps. If I got it wrong or said the wrong thing, he would say so. What we needed was family therapy. What he got was Cognitive Behaviour Therapy CBT. I'm sure it works for some, but Andrew seemed to come out more confused than anything else and as I hadn't any idea of what was going on, I couldn't help him.

On one occasion at the last minute he said I really can't go, I'm not well enough and I can't go through all that. As I was going in to town anyway, I called to tell the psychologist that he wasn't going and she wanted to see Ron and me. She had lots of questions, but when I asked her

ANDREW'S STORY

anything, she said she couldn't tell me, patient confidentiality! This was my son's welfare we were talking about! I told her that he was isolated living with us and needed someone to take him out to social meetings of some sort, where he could meet people like himself. I asked when there were sessions in the art room that I had noticed in Park House. There aren't any, we don't use it any more! We can't afford a teacher! (I remember many years ago my father said to me, 'when a business is in trouble, they sack the tea lady')!

The next time we met the psychologist she started pumping me for information I told her, if she wanted to know ask Andrew, parent confidentiality! This wasn't working out.

Andrew asked if he could go back to Bristol but that doctor had moved on to a different part of their service, pity!

Chapter 14

Round and round and round!

Although we had the Council's housing report we didn't have the file notes their opinion was based on and so I asked for them. We were told that our solicitor had everything. I said we had looked at the reports he had, but wanted to see what they were based on. The file was sent but I was convinced it was not complete.

With the intervention of the Access Officer and many months later, we were eventually given all the information we had asked for. There was a running day report which we and the solicitor hadn't seen. It was five pages long and, in my opinion, quite damning.

There was reference to the Liverpool episode and how disappointed we were with the visit as we had found the professor abrasive. It said that I felt someone had told him about Andrew's addiction to methadone as we had not informed him of it. The note said she asked why someone would do that and I am supposed to have said, I thought someone was trying to hinder Andrew's case. This was based on some truth, but a certain spin had been put on it and it would have been better left out of her housing report, I couldn't see what it had to do with homelessness.

There was reference to receiving a phone call from Dr. Morkane regarding her letter to the PCT re-submitting the medical problems. He asked her about the homeless procedure and it was discussed at length. She explained how she investigated claims and the factors taken into account. The guidance from the GP had been returned marked 'not vulnerable'. She couldn't understand why Andrew was claiming top rate Disability Living Allowance when his GP said he wasn't vulnerable. As Dr. Morkane was advising the Council on behalf of the PCT, I was surprised that he had to ask her about procedures, I thought he would have known them!

The record then showed that Dr. Morkane contacted her again saying he had spoken to the GP and they stood by the decision that Andrew was not vulnerable. We couldn't find the letter from the GP in the file and I asked for a copy, but we didn't get it!

Dr. Morkane spoke to the investigator again and told her that Andrew's current property was suitable for him, although he had never been there. She had told Dr. Morkane that it was actually owned by Andrew's parents! It was them that had given him notice which would make him homeless! (I complained to the Information Commissioner that no permission had been given to share that information, but it was not upheld).

Again it was stated that Dr. Morkane didn't understand the system until she had explained it. She said she would be consulting with the fraud department over non-payment of housing benefit!

There was a copy of the form on which Dr. Morkane based his opinion. It was sent to the GP to fill in and had just two tick boxes for him to complete.

The first;

Has s/he any medical condition which interferes with mobility. Yes/ No.

The second.

Has s/he any mental health problems or condition which would put he/her into the category of vulnerability. Yes/No.

And that was it! That's what people with serious health problems are assessed on. This is what decisions are made on as to whether people should live on the streets or be socially housed. Two tick boxes!

ANDREW'S STORY

The report then referred to me asking the social worker for a referral to a psychiatric nurse, initially the social worker said she would refer him, then came back to say, see your GP. Apparently I had told her that I didn't have any 'faith' in the GP! Then the report said the doctor had refused to refer him. I don't know where that came from as Andrew was too afraid to ask him for one.

The social worker was contacted and she told the investigator that Andrew's domestic help had been withdrawn and, "The illness itself does not make him vulnerable, but the way he deals with it does'.

It was recorded that I had told the social worker Andrew had lost weight in the last couple of months due to his illness, which was true! It goes up and down like a yo-yo sometimes.

From the PSN

'Hi All,
I haven't been on in a while due to my husband being ill again, his weight has now dropped from nearly eighteen stone to seven stone eight. He had a week in hospital for more tests and is due to have an operation in the next three months, we hope it will help him.

I was really wondering how many people with chronic Pancreatitis or any type of Pancreatitis could actually work or even be expected to work.

My husband did manage quite well at first but is obviously unable to work now and I doubt he will ever be able to again. His employer had refused ill health retirement twice now.

Hi,
I'm so lucky in that I am a software developer so I can work from home if I'm not well enough to go in. My attitude is that if my pain and afflictions allow me to manage to walk, I will go to work. It really annoys me when colleagues ring up and have the day off on the sick with a cold or sore back, but then, our pain threshold is much higher than normal people.

Pringy'

And.

'The problem with Pancreatitis is that it has such variable levels of progression and disabling effects. Some people have a worse time with it than others; there are no 'one fit all' situations. I've been lucky (it's all relative) and so far have not suffered as badly as others on this forum. Fitness for work is only something the sufferer can judge in conjunction with their doctors.'

ANDREW'S STORY

'Thanks for your replies. He is having his gall bladder removed and part of his pancreas, the tube that leads to his stomach and also part of his bowel and intestine. He has 'Groove Pancreatitis' quite a rare form of chronic Pancreatitis. At the first hospital he was in, it was only the second case they had ever seen. He has been referred to another hospital now and it is the ninth case they have seen.

He should have had a feeding tube fitted before Christmas to stop the weight loss but they can't get it down as the tube to his stomach has totally shut off, they don't want a neck drip due to the risk of infection, so he just has to wait for the operation, I hope it works!'

And from New Zealand

'I'm retired, age 50 and enjoyed life and travel immensely, living off superannuation and some commissions which I continued to receive, until that day when I was struck with the most horrific pain known to man. From that day work became impossible for me. I now pay people to mow my lawn and do the jobs that I once enjoyed doing myself.

I am certainly capable of administrative work, brain over brawn, but cannot guarantee that at any given time I will be fit enough to carry out any task. Believe me, when you are in pain you are not capable of doing much whether it be mental or physical.

Prior to my operation I spent thirteen periods in hospital in twelve months and lost weight, from 65 kg to 45kg, I have just managed to get back to 52kg. I have no Pancreas at all, so why when I lift anything do I have such pain?

Your husband is not on his own not being fit for work, there are many like him. His greatest concern, I imagine, is how to recover some of his weight. Losing weight weakens you and makes it so much harder to recover. Give him my regards and assure him he is not an odd one out.

Employers don't understand this condition (nor do a very large number of medical professionals). If you had told the employers that it was cancer they would have been most sympathetic and understanding. Tell them it's Pancreatitis and they will say, Yeah OK, he will he back at work next week then! RAY'

The Council investigator had spoken with the DLA and asked for an answer to her letter commenting on the new evidence from the GP, which said that Andrew was not medically vulnerable. DLA said they would order over the file from the store which would take a few days. They told her that the original claim for DLA was refused but this went to appeal and was overturned.

The notes said Dr. Morkane had written a letter telling the DLA that Andrew was not entitled to DLA and that the letter would be put on the DLA file for the next application when the present award ran out! I asked Dr. Morkane for a copy of that letter but he could not find it and didn't remember writing it!

DLA were phoned again and 'Sam' said they had no papers from the appeal and so could not see why the appeal was upheld. But it did look as though Andrew was not vulnerable according to Dr. Morkane's letter. She would speak to a senior adviser.

The next entry said, she spoke to Sam again who had spoken with a decision maker, they confirmed that the award was for five years. Again Sam said Dr. Morkane's letter indicated that Andrew was not vulnerable, but Sam could not identify why the appeal was upheld. The Council investigator then asked if the new evidence would be put forward when the next review of DLA took place. Sam said they would be aware of this and the decision maker would assess the information. She was in agreement that medical guidance which stated that Andrew was not medical vulnerable, did not coincide with payment of DLA. Sam was unable to answer why this was possible.

These notes are what the Council relied on when sending a witness statement to be used in Court! There's something very wrong here.

The Council were asked for a copy of the letter referred to in their file notes, the one from the GP. They replied (again) that I had everything in the file and suggested that I ask the GP. I did and he said he didn't have Andrew's notes any more, ask his new GP!

*   *   *

I wrote to Social Services asking for a short simple letter explaining that it was a change of their policy that triggered withdrawal of Andrew's domestic help. He had not done anything wrong as the wording of the housing report implied. I wanted to send the letter to the council to explain the situation and to put the record straight. I also asked on what information Trisha based her opinion of Andrew's illness, "That the illness itself would not make him vulnerable, but the way he let it affect him would." How many other clients had she with Hereditary Childhood Pancreatitis? Who had advised her?

ANDREW'S STORY

Six weeks after I wrote to Social Services, I received a reply from the area manager. In it she 'reviewed' Andrew's case and social services involvement, the letter was a page and a half long. Almost all the facts referred to were wrong,

'Andrew used his support worker to ferry him about and that service was withdrawn. His needs are predominantly around budgeting and social skills/interaction.

I understand that he has another support worker who is assisting with these needs and which may lead to other community access opportunities.

I can understand that you found the letter from Council difficult, but I think this is partly due to the language they use. I cannot pass comment on their mentioning Andrew's domestic care but I emphasise that our policy did not change. Andrew was receiving a service for which he was ineligible and in any case it was agreed with him that it was inappropriate to meet his needs'.

It ended with;

'By definition in the general sense of the word, many people Social Services comes into contact with are 'vulnerable'. However, both the Borough Council and Social Services have clear policy and definitions around what is meant by vulnerable.

The Council have, after consultation with Andrew's GP, decided he does not meet their medical vulnerability criteria and our definition of a vulnerable adult is 'an individual who is unable to care for themselves by virtue of old age, mental or physical incapacity, sensory loss or learning disability/difficulties, or for any reason is unable to protect him or herself against significant harm or exploitation. Andrew clearly does not fit these criteria.'

I replied that all I asked for was a simple letter saying Andrew did nothing wrong when his one hour a week help was withdrawn. That her 'review' was incorrect in many aspects and I expressed my astonishment that a person who could not digest food without intervention and had all the health problems that he had, was not considered to be disabled!

Trisha should have informed us about the 'duty slot' at Park House but there was no reference to that or to where Trish's information came from. I said that her letter took our breath away and I didn't want to hear from her again....

I wrote to the complaints officer asking what they based their assessment on. I explained that I had asked for a simple letter but received a long inaccurate review which was offensive to us. I asked for a copy of social services policy and to see the file again. There was much prevarication over the file and we were asked why did we want to see it again? I explained that I now had reason to believe it had been 'combed' before we had seen it. That was denied. Eventually, they came here to our house with the file, it took two of them. I let Andrew read it as he was a faster reader that I am and it did seem much fatter than before. They said it just had more letters added to it as they came in. Andrew was in fact now slow at reading. Was it medication that slowed him down?

It is quite intimidating, two strangers sitting in silence while you try to concentrate on something. After one hour they made to move saying they had another appointment to attend. It was 1 pm. I thought it must be lunch they wanted. I asked for another appointment at which they seemed most put out! We had seen the file! I explained we had day running notes from the borough council, which contained pages sent from Social Services, so far we hadn't found any of them in the file, one hour was not long enough. "Oh, day sheets are kept in another file; you didn't say you wanted to see them!" It was information that had never been offered before! They said they would send a photo copy, they did but I'm still not convinced we had the entire file! We really wanted to see what contact there had been with the doctor, but there was little reference in the day notes. The hand writing was difficult to read and the notes were printed back to back and out of date order, it was mostly impossible to follow them, they won in the end!

There was no answer from Social Services to my letter of complaint, so I wrote again, this time they gave an apology for not acknowledging receipt of the first letter but assuring me, given the nature of my concerns that it had been passed to the Head of Primary Care Service. The complaints manager said he understood that she was meeting the staff concerned and would contact me. I was sent a leaflet called Fair Access for All; this was in response to asking for a copy of their policy document.

Later I received a quarter page report with an apology for the delay. It said the language used throughout the area manager's letter was appropriate and professional and they could not agree the letter was offensive. Therefore, they were unable to support my complaint. However, if I was not satisfied they would meet me to discuss it further.

I asked for a meeting and heard nothing more until I reminded them.
Then, we did receive a letter saying that it **was** a change of policy and that social services no longer supplied home help! They also said that I expressed a different opinion of matters about

some aspects of Social Services involvement. Not
being sure what that meant I decided that the
letter was not suitable to send to the Borough
Council!

Eventually a meeting was arranged and I said that
all I asked for was a short simple letter saying that
Andrew had done nothing wrong when his home
help was stopped. What was wrong with that? I
was told that they had done that, but I said the
letter was long inaccurate and not fit for purpose!
I couldn't send that. I also said that he was
disabled and to say he wasn't has offended us
greatly.

They asked me to suggest the wording, which I
did, but they didn't like my wording, we negotiated
and the wording was agreed, eventually I received
a suitable letter to send to the Council. It had
taken many, many months.

After this, there followed months of exchanges
between the complaints officer and myself
regarding the content of the area manager's letter.
I explained to them why what she had written was
simply wrong and I gave evidence to support my
account, a year later we received an apology, but
the area manager was not disciplined!

*   *   *

In 2003 we wrote to the Primary Care Trust asking how the Director of Public Health could inform the Council that Andrew, with five major health problems was not medically vulnerable. I asked for a definition of what is medical vulnerability? No answer was forthcoming and I had to write again, doesn't anyone answer letters without being reminded? This time I made an official complaint saying that the PCT should put its house in order so that sick people do not have to make complaints about doctors. They knew about the poor performance of the Practise in question and did nothing about it. Eventually a letter came back vindicating their actions and saying if we were not satisfied we could complain to the Healthcare Commission...

I wrote to the Healthcare Commission, by now it was 2004 and their answer was that I had sent enough evidence for them to investigate our complaint but all their investigators were busy. They didn't know how long it would be before they could look at the matter. I wrote to their Chief Executive asking, as they were not able to tell me when they would look into our case, could I go straight to the Health and Social Care Ombudsman? I also said that I thought their office was under funded. My son had already tried to commit suicide and I thought it important that this was dealt with soon.

ANDREW'S STORY

The response was that we must go through the Healthcare Commission route of the complaints procedure first, before going on to the Healthcare Ombudsman and the matter would be dealt with as soon as possible. Our name came to the top of the waiting list in three months and the investigation began. I was asked for further information and letters. By now the file was getting quite fat! I had been a bit careless with information and had lost some letters at the start of all this. How could I have known it would spiral to this extent and that it would matter? Now I had learnt my lesson and tried to mend my ways and be methodical and very careful how I filed things! How I wished I had kept a diary.

A phone call from the investigator told us that they could not look at how anything has affected anyone personally, only the way in which information was collected. More letters and answers were asked for and then we waited.

I received a letter apologising for the delay in the report, it was because the investigator was trying to obtain a copy of the judgement from the court and was waiting for a transcription to be carried out. I said I could give her one if it was important and it was duly sent off, a weighty document! I didn't think to wonder at the time why she wanted it; I just wanted all this over and finished with.

Some months later the outcome of the initial review arrived for us to comment on. It was three pages long and said that our complaint had raised three issues.

1. The process by which the PCT, through the Director of Public Health, provided a medical opinion to the local authority's housing department in relation to an assessment of medical vulnerability.

I have decided to ask the PCT to take further action about this aspect of your complaint because the assessment request form that GP's are asked to complete is too restrictive.

Under the Housing Act 1996, local council's only have to ensure housing is available if they consider the applicant to be vulnerable. The definition of vulnerability is not precise. The PCT process has remained virtually unchanged for a number of years. A letter of guidance with some changes has been sent to all GPs and I enclose a copy for your information. The form will be amended by the PCT.

I have sought advice from the Office of the Deputy Prime Minister.
Their advice is that physical disability or long term acute illness, such as those defined by the

ANDREW'S STORY

Disability Discrimination Act 1995 should also be considered.

(The report didn't say that if a person is defined by the Disability Discrimination Act there was no need to take advice, as that person was deemed to be vulnerable in housing terms anyway, so taking advice was unnecessary).

Whilst I appreciate that this is too late to help your son I hope that the changes I have recommended will ensure that when the local authority is considering applications in the future, it will be able to make a fully informed decision.

(The guidance given to the Healthcare Commission from the ODPM seemed to be on housing allocation, not homelessness, judging by what the investigator said on the phone. It was not in line with the information given to me by Shelter).

2. The PCT was aware of the reputation and standard of the service of the GP practice that Andrew was registered with at the time and therefore should not have provided an opinion based on advice received from that GP.

(It didn't say why the PCT hadn't approached the consultants involved with his care, as I had asked them to do.)

I have decided not to take further action on this, as the PCT have procedures in place to monitor this.

(They may have procedures in place but it didn't help us! I asked if they took the previous administrations records into account since this PCT had only been in place for six to nine months. No answer).

3. The PCT ignored numerous requests by you for information.

I have decided not to take further action on this issue because much of the information you requested was data protected and confidential. It would have been helpful if they had told you that at an earlier date.

The PCT apologised for not acknowledging your letters and staff have been reminded of the need to respond promptly.

(They still don't)!

If you are still dissatisfied you can appeal to the Health Service Ombudsman. If you have any questions about any aspect of this letter, please don't hesitate to contact me.

ANDREW'S STORY

I spoke to the lady who made this report and told her that I thought the wrong guidance had been given by the ODPM; it was allocations advice, not homeless advice. We discussed it; her version was different to Shelter's and she asked for a copy which I put in the post.

I phoned the ODPM and asked who monitored their guidance on homelessness and was told there were no guidance notes on homelessness, I assured her there were. They would get back to me but nothing happened. I phoned again. The lady on the phone didn't know anything, but would look into my query and phone me back, needless to say, I didn't hear from her again.

A week later there was another letter from the Healthcare Commission saying among other things, that further information was on the web site of the ODPM, it sets out the Homelessness Code of Guidance. This was after she had made her report which she did not change. They had all missed the point, where a disability is covered by the Disability Discrimination Act, there is medical vulnerability and where there is medical vulnerability they must help homeless disabled people!

This whole nightmare could have been avoided if everyone had followed the guidance that, where disability is covered by the DDA, (diabetes is covered), they do not have to seek more advice. They can if they wish, but what is the point, the guidance says they are vulnerable. Why waste resources if it's not necessary. But if authority can get away with it, then precious resources are saved by not having to house a vulnerable sick person! Authority is also told to follow the spirit of the Law.

I wasn't satisfied with the Healthcare Commission report and as advised by them, I filled in the next form and complained to the Healthcare Ombudsman. I received an answer telling me to go back to the Healthcare Commission as the first step was not completed regarding the new form and the PCT.

'I am therefore of the view that the best way ahead is for you write (English?) to the Healthcare Commission and ask that they consider your complaint again. If following that you remain dissatisfied, please write to us again'. That from the screening department at the Ombudsman Office! I wasn't sure what nationality the lady was, my observation was that I didn't think it was English.

And so we waited for the PCT to make the alterations to the form that the Healthcare Commission had asked for, before we could proceed to the Ombudsman. Four months later and still waiting!   I wrote to the Healthcare Commission that we had heard nothing, they wrote to the PCT who apologised but they were 'consulting with the borough council'. She gave them a month to make an interim amendment in consultation with Shelter, and we should receive a copy. Her letter was copied to the Strategic Health Authority.

A month later the PCT wrote to the Commission acknowledging the time taken in complying with their direction.

'You will appreciate that this process involves the local authority as well as the Primary Care Trust and therefore the time scale for the review has not been wholly within the Trust's control. I nevertheless accept that the delay has been regrettable and apologise for this shortcoming.

You have spoken to Dr. Morkane and clarified the issues in relation to assessing medical vulnerability for housing. As noted, assessments vary significantly between PCT's as do the questions asked to ascertain medical conditions and vulnerability.

The form used by us has been in use for several years and was initiated under the former Health Authority. The letter now used is similar to that used by other PCT's in Somerset, but not all.

The letter has now been further modified and I enclose a copy of the revised format. I confirm that the amendments reflect comments made by Shelter.

I have, as requested, copied this letter to Andrew but would emphasise that the letter only applies to people covered by the homeless legislation. As you know he is not now homeless but is on the housing list.

I can confirm that we remain willing to review his priority points on the housing list should we be asked to do so by the housing department.'

This letter astonished me. How can the PCT have input to housing points? On enquiry, Shelter said, the PCT had **not** consulted with them as the Healthcare Commission had requested. They had **not** been asked to comment and had **not** seen the new form. I supplied them with a copy; their comment was that they still had 'fundamental problems' with the form in its new modified form.

My children had been teaching me a new vocabulary and with their education I thought this response was a load of crap!

My next letter to the PCT said their letter to the Healthcare Commission raised more questions.

ANDREW'S STORY

Healthcare Commission could not look at the way these issues had affected Andrew personally they said, only the way in which the PCT collected information. I asked who had been updating them on Andrew's current housing situation as I thought that was data protected information. They were correct that Andrew wasn't homeless now as we had taken him in and provided a roof over his head. We find it unbelievable that with his major health problems that the PCT say he is not medically vulnerable. I asked what medical vulnerability is if five major health problems are not.

I assured the Chief Executive that Shelter had not been consulted on the format of the form and that if the form had been modified, as they had promised the previous year, Andrew would not have been caught by its short comings.

We expressed astonishment that they will review housing points. Wasn't that the responsibility of the housing department, how could they have input to that?

Two weeks later Mr. Colgan acknowledged my letter saying he would respond in ten days. A month later I wrote saying how disappointed I was not to hear from him. Then a reply apologising for the delay and saying they had been in consultation with the Council.

'You will appreciate that the position regarding Andrew's application has been fully reviewed as part of the NHS complaints procedure and I do not intend to revisit those issues again.

On that basis, I have nothing further to add to previous comments made by the PCT'.

The Healthcare Commission letters had all been copied to the Strategic Health Authority, so I wrote to them,

'Can you please tell me how a PCT can say that a person with no Pancreas and with 5 major health problems, mal-absorption, steatorrhoea, chronic pain syndrome, diabetes and depression can be described as not being medically vulnerable'?

An answer (in two days!) *'The Strategic Health Authority does not have responsibility for investigating complaints against a PCT and are unable to comment on this matter'.* I wonder what they do at the Strategic Health Authority.

I wrote back, *'I am aware that the Strategic Health Authority does not have responsibility for investigating complaints, but according to their web site responsibilities do include, 'management performance, holding PCT's to account and improving standards'*

ANDREW'S STORY

Again I asked what qualifies as medically vulnerable in their terms. I thought they would like to know how this PCT deals with these situations. The response was a phone call from the Assistant Director of Public Affairs, he reiterated they will not get involved, they have no opinion. The phone call was followed by a letter from their chief executive Sir Ian Carruthers saying, "I hope this has clarified the matter for you?"

Again I asked myself, what does the Strategic Health Authority do? It certainly costs the tax payer a lot of money. In order to save money perhaps it should be done away with? The money could then be spent on the front line instead of closing beds and departments and cutting down on help for people in need. If we close down Strategic Health, what ever that is, we could spend the money on people who need services which we apparently can't afford!

*   *   *

I phoned the Healthcare Commissioner investigator who said that if I wanted a further investigation I should, as a first step, tell the PCT that I was not satisfied with their response. I said it was all part of the original complaint. "No, the case was now closed; this would be a new complaint." I wrote again to the PCT saying this was now a further complaint. How can they have input to housing points which is Council responsibility. They had not consulted Shelter as they said they had. They had still not told me what medical vulnerability is. The situation is not satisfactory and again they said they had nothing further to add.

I asked for a copy of the file the PCT held, that had anything to do with me or my son. It came several weeks later. The PAL's officer at the PCT had found five other complaints, but we had been told there were no concerns over the practice.

I went back to the Healthcare Investigation unit and I was told there would be another long wait before there could be any investigation, the waiting list is even longer now! That was unfair I protested it was really all part of the previous case. Take it to the Health and Parliamentary Ombudsman they suggested, but I explained that I had already done that and the case was sent back to them for review! I contacted the Ombudsman's office and they wanted confirmation that the case had been through the Healthcare 'review' procedure! This is just like ping pong, bat and ball, this could go on for years! Little did I know that it would!

*   *   *

ANDREW'S STORY

Back to Healthcare Commission with a plea for some help that I could understand, it was all very confusing....The review was complete and I could proceed to the Ombudsman with the first complaint. The second complaint was awaiting investigation. In the mean time.........

I wrote to the Office of the Deputy Prime Minister in April asking who monitors their guidelines on homelessness and what happens to Local Authorities who do not follow them. The reply was a page long expressing sadness at the problems my son has but telling me that they cannot get involved in individual cases. It told me that Councils must publish their allocation schemes and suggested that we go to the Citizens Advice Bureau. No answer to my question!

In May I asked my MP if he could find out who monitored government guidelines on homelessness. He wrote to the Minister for Housing and Planning and she replied. This time a page and half of good advice on housing although they could not comment on individual cases, advice on what local authorities must publish about their procedures, sadness at the health problems my son had and suggested that we go to the CAB, but no answer to my question!

I emailed the Housing and Planning Minister's office thanking them for their answer to my MP, but saying the question I asked was who monitors the guidelines, would they please tell me? No answer!

I phoned the ODPM and asked who monitors their guidelines on homelessness? This time I was told that my request for information would be forwarded on for reply. Nothing happened, there was no reply.

My MP and I agreed that I should make a complaint to the Parliamentary Ombudsman and he got the form for me saying, fill it in and I will send it back for you, which we did.

The Parliamentary Ombudsman replied with a review of my case with the Healthcare Commission, nothing to do with guidelines published by the ODPM! The letter said there had been difficulty in securing a response from the PCT in the issues referred back to them, but understood they expected a response shortly. He suggested that I go back to the Healthcare Commission and ask them to consider my complaint again! No answer to my question, who monitors the ODPM guidelines!

I emailed the author saying that I had tried to phone, but there was no one in the office to take my call. I asked for an explanation of why he had reviewed the Healthcare Commission case, when

ANDREW'S STORY

my letter was about information given or not given, by the ODPM. The question is who monitors your guidelines? That has nothing to do with the Healthcare Commission; it is your office who should deal with this! My last sentence was what do we have to do to obtain justice?

I received a phone call saying that he and several colleges had misread my letter, his colleague would write to me!

We had an acknowledgement and an apology for the 'cross over' of my Healthcare Service complaint with the complaint to the ODPM! They would enter my complaint on their register, and nine months after I first started asking for information; we were on another waiting list, again! Well, if they can't sort out their files and understand their system and what is happening, what hope is there for me to understand what's going on?

In November 2005 we were informed that the case (about the ODPM) had been allocated to the Parliamentary Ombudsman's investigator. After Christmas with nothing happening, I made further enquiries and was told that an investigator was about to be appointed to my complaint! I really am confused now it's all getting so complicated, what with one department seemingly playing me off against another.

By the end of January the investigator phoned to say she had finished her initial enquiry and had found nothing wrong with the information given to the Healthcare Commission by the ODPM. I told her that the Healthcare Commission had been given housing allocations information, not homeless guidance. She asked me for a copy of the papers I had been given by Shelter. When I received a copy of her report, the last paragraph said, she had read the papers I had submitted but considered them to mean the same thing and so she had not altered her decision. There was no mention of, who monitors the guidelines! If allocations and homelessness guidelines are the same, why are there two guidelines? I asked for a review!

She seemed a little put out that I should question her report and ask for it to be looked at again, we went on to the next stage of the complaint procedure (regarding the ODPM) and were back on another waiting list, again.

                    *   *   *

Back on the Healthcare Commission front, second complaint, a two page letter with eight paragraphs from the 'Complaints Team' entitled: 'Your request for independent review', arrived. There was an apology for the delay in responding; (only three months, that's good for them)! It was just an amazing document!

1. Continued failure to acknowledge receipt or provide a timely response.

It is unclear if this has been raised as a formal complaint! If so provide copies of correspondence.
(I did, nothing happened! You have copies of the letters).

2. Explanation of PCT's view that your son is not medially vulnerable.

I understand that these issues have been referred to the Parliament Ombudsman and therefore it would not be appropriate for me to consider them further.
(There should be an answer in the Healthcare report then, please direct me to it)!

3. The PCT's position regarding your son's DLA.

The benefit process is not an area that falls within the NHS complaints procedure. However, the statement that the PCT will comment if asked appears to be perfectly reasonable to me.
(If benefit procedures fall outside NHS, why did Dr. Morkane have an opinion and write to the DLA, what are you going to do about it)?

4. Further assessment by the PCT.

Further assessment would have been against criteria set down by the local authority. I would expect the PCT to decline if they did not consider they had the appropriate expertise.
(Please tell me where that information came from. How do they know about the criteria of the Local authority)?

5. Why the PAL's officer left the PCT.

That falls outside the NHS complaints procedure. (I expect the reason the PAL's officer 'left' was that she got the situation right and that was an embarrassment to the PCT).

6. The information provided by the Healthcare Commission regarding the doctor involved with the assessment.

(The PCT said there were no concerns about the performance of the doctor and any action taken was not as a result of the complaint. There seems to be no understanding, the PCT gave wrong information to the Healthcare Commission. There were complaints, at least five. I asked that the PCT should put its own house in order, they didn't. What are you going to do about it)?

7. The PCT has not provided a copy of the amended form.

The PCT's letter dated 15th August says it provided a copy to you. I recommend you request a further copy from the PCT.
(I recommend you read the Healthcare Commission's letter of the 9th August 2005. There was only an interim form and that was never approved by Shelter. There was never a final form)!

8. Previous review of your complaint. This is currently being reviewed and it would not be appropriate to comment at this time.

I finished my letter to them, 'No one takes responsibility and we are just left to get on with it! Why can't someone just say sorry?

There was an acknowledgement to this letter and nothing more, so I phoned their office. I was told the hold up was that the Healthcare Commission was waiting for a response from the PCT. They were expecting it any day now. Two weeks later I phoned again and enquired why were we still waiting, in conversation I was told there had been six calls to the PCT and it had elicited nothing! They had now written to them.

Brenda Prentice

Five months after first writing there was an answer! None of my comments were considered and the review for both issues (I thought there were eight, plus four others in all) was closed!

I asked for a review and in three days an answer, 'there was nothing further for us to review'. I complained to their Chief Executive Anna Walker, again.

Her response was:

'I understand your frustration at what must seem like a bureaucratic approach and the lack of a system which can look at your concerns as a whole across the actions of the PCT and the Council. Unfortunately, we have to act within the powers given to us in our legislation. This means we cannot consider issues relating to how the local council has performed its functions: concerns about information request or concerns and complaints about healthcare providers that have not first been raised with the provider concerned'.

And so it went on for one and a half pages. It ended with,

'I am sorry that you need to take different aspects of your concerns to different agencies. We have attempted to identify who you need to contact on particular issues and I hope this will be helpful'.

ANDREW'S STORY

I wrote back, '*sadly whoever advised you, had not answered my questions. Shelter still advises me that no one has been in contact with them, please advise the name of the person you think has consulted with Shelter, they would like to know.*

Why do the PCT say they have control over housing points?

What is medical vulnerability if five major problems are not?
If fault was found with the PCT and it was, why are we told, 'we cannot look at how it has affected anyone personally, when a solicitor says you can'?'

I ended up with;

'*I thought all these departments were set up to help the public. I have revised my opinion*'.

*　　　　　*
*

In January 2006, a report came from the Parliamentary and Health Ombudsman. This one regarding information from the ODPM given to the Healthcare Commission.

The review said that the information given was correct! That's right, information given was correct, but it should have been information on homelessness, not information on allocations! I was told it meant the same thing! So why are there two lots of guidance notes, one on homelessness and one on allocations? They are different and if read it is obvious they do not mean the same thing! This system is not set up for people to win!

*   *   *

Another letter arrived from the Parliamentary and Health Service Ombudsman, 'this letter is my report to you of the results of the investigations and my findings'. This refers to the first complaint, (I think). In the eight pages there were thirty three references and none were in our favour.

'As the PCT no longer exists as a distinct entity, I can see no merit in making any criticisms of or recommendations to the PCT'.

(So the new PCT can't learn from any mistakes made by the old PCT. I should have known).

To my question why has the PCT failed to answer why is my son not considered medically vulnerable? There was an answer.

ANDREW'S STORY

'Neither the PCT nor the Commission can determine whether a person is medically vulnerable in relation to housing legislation. Therefore I do not criticise them for not answering your question. Indeed they would have been acting beyond their role had they attempted to do so. I should add that the Ombudsman too cannot answer your question'.

(But the PCT did carry out an assessment so they must have an answer to the question. Why else would they have made the assessment? Council took advice from the PCT who said he is not vulnerable and the Judge said; where advice is taken it must be reliable!

So who is responsible for this almighty cock up? I simply can't get my head round all this shifting about. It seems to me that each authority tells it like they want it to be! Someone must have a definitive answer to what is medical vulnerability! If there is no answer, why is the question asked in the first place?)

Their conclusion.

'I hope that you will be reassured that your concerns about the actions of the PCT and the Commission have now been thoroughly and independently reviewed, and that no major short comings have been identified. The PCT is no

*longer involved in the process of assessing
medical vulnerability and that seems to me to be a
good thing. They were, in effect, acting only as
messengers and direct contact between those
doing the assessment (the council) and applicants'
clinicians. It will prevent problems of this nature
occurring again'.*
(So why are Nowmedical being recommended by
the PCT, they are not the 'applicants clinician'! So
'problems of this nature,' will happen again!)

I asked for a review!

*   *   *

An article from Manchester Hospital Trust: A
Decade of Research.

*'There is little effective treatment for Chronic
Pancreatitis. This disease causes severe pain
that can only be controlled by narcotic analgesics
– morphine and pethidine. These addictive drugs
cause personality and behaviour changes such
that patients are unable to hold on to their jobs,
they become demoralized, family life is broken up
and there are all the costs of social security
payments to maintain them'.*

The Manchester Trust recognises the difficulties
associated with this life shattering disease.
What's wrong with our PCT doing the same? They

are all driving me crazy with their inability to answer straight forward questions. They are masters at avoiding the issue!
I wonder which university offers degrees in that subject!

Chapter 15

Calm before the Storm.

Our entire life now seemed to revolve round
Andrew and his problems. It was becoming
difficult for us to take a holiday; this is the time of
our life that we should be able to please ourselves
what we do and when we do it! We have worked
hard all our lives, this should be retirement. Many
of our neighbours in the village, who are now
retired, were taking long cruises; one had just
been round the world! Another had been to the
Galapagos Islands and on to South America! And
yet another visited the West Indies!

We talked about holidays and thought we might
leave Andrew for a day or two but not for longer.
He was so depressed I felt it would not be safe to
leave him longer. Between the three of us we
decided that another river cruise might be nice
and Andrew would come with us. We studied the
brochures and after a long discussion we decided
to 'do' the River Douro in Portugal which comes
down from Spain. There was a day out from the
boat by coach to Salamanca where April had been
at university for six months. She had always said
'you must visit; it is such a beautiful city'. The
thing about a cruise is that if Andrew had a bad
day and just wanted to stay in bed and sleep he

could, while we can do things and still keep an eye on him.

We flew from Bristol to Porto, as journeys go, it was not too arduous for Andrew and we were soon on the boat. Unlike the Rhine and Moselle cruise that we had been on before, the boat was not tied up in town but some way out on the other side of the river. There seemed to be nothing of much interest to see apart from traffic going over a very new and modern bridge. There was a very steep hill to climb the other way into a very nondescript village. We thought we would not be there for long and made the best of it.

The next day we left our berth and started down river, or should that be up? The boat and crew were mainly French as were most of the passengers! As my French is nil I relied on Ron and Andrew or the translations which followed all announcements to know what was going on. The boat was new and very well appointed and the food, being a French owned boat, was good but then, so was the food on the Rhine cruise! The crew worked hard to serve and entertain us. Andrew never made it to breakfast or lunch but sometimes came to dinner. Otherwise I took him a tray with what I thought he might be able to eat. The trip was a little disappointing, with few towns to visit along the river edge and we didn't want to do many of the coach trips that were laid on for us.

The trip to Salamanca left the boat at 7am and Andrew was up at 6.30! As the coach didn't depart until 7.45, he did wonder why he had made the effort, but he did want to see the town that April had spoken of so many times. After we got started, the tour made good use of the day and we saw many tourist attractions with time for lunch in the square and a well earned rest... Andrew was exhausted!

On our return from the holiday I wrote to the Local Government Ombudsman on Andrew's behalf and complained about the housing decision. Andrew wrote his own statement and attached it. Five pages long, it took a lot of effort and concentration on his part.

He stated how long he had been ill and that the housing advice was contradictory and he didn't know what to do for the best when he couldn't pay the mortgage on his new flat. A Social Services report had said that he needed a stable environment, it had been ignored and he had moved four times in three years as there was no help available to him. His housing benefit application had not been determined, he could not pay the rent to his parents after his money ran out and that would threaten their own home as they had mortgaged it to help him. He paid £800 a year for his insulin pump sundries and now his parents would have to pay for that as he had no money.

The Occupational Therapist said he should have a shower but the effort of organising it was too much and when he told Social Services he would not continue with its installation, they didn't pass the message on to the Council. The Councils report shouldn't say, we didn't tell them, we did!

After his money ran out, his Piper Emergency line was sent back as he could not pay the phone bill. He felt he owed money to everyone; he didn't answer the phone, open the door or letters. He spiralled down into deep depression and eventually was made bankrupt. The Council sent the Bailiffs even though they knew that his parents had a Power of Attorney but parents were not kept informed. Many letters were sent to the Council asking for advice but they were never answered.

We had asked for sheltered accommodation for a disabled person but were told there isn't any for people under sixty. We asked for appropriate accommodation for disabled people on grounds of medical vulnerability and this was turned down, he was told he is not medically vulnerable.

The Council say they have a letter from the doctor saying he is not vulnerable but, although we have asked, we have not seen a copy of it and don't think it exists. The Council told Shelter they would not use the housing form again and then used it for his application. The Council told the DLA that Dr. Morkane said he is not vulnerable and not entitled to DLA and the DLA say the benefit is no measure of housing need.

Andrew said that Harry, from the council, was to have sorted out his housing benefit and hadn't. That the Housing Authority are expected to act in the spirit of the law and take into consideration abnormal expenditure by clients, he did pay for the sundries of his insulin pump but it was not taken into consideration. The fact that continuing vomiting puts up the cost of a grocery bill was not considered, even though at one time the Social Services gave Andrew a £10 grocery voucher as he was penniless and without food.

He now had to live with his parents and it wasn't fair to them, he was isolated and had no transport. The taxi fare from hospital can be anything from £14 to £40 depending on the time of day or night, none of which was considered.

It took Andrew several days to complete the statement and I was very proud that he managed it. Constant chronic pain saps energy and concentration, it leaves victims weak and weary, so the statement was a great achievement for him.

ANDREW'S STORY

We waited for an Ombudsman investigator to be appointed to deal with our case and eventually we came to the top of the waiting list. They could not look at anything that has been to Court but could look at other peripheral issues. He listed from Andrews's statement what he thought he could look at and wrote to the Council.

I also explained to the Ombudsman that I had asked to see the information which had been used to make their housing report. I felt that it wasn't easy to extract this from the Council and I had to keep insisting until I got it. It took a long time.

Many months later we had a copy of the council's response to the Ombudsman for us to comment on if we wished. Basically they rejected all the complaints.

I then gave as much information as I had to support our claim and I thought it did discredit what the Council had to say. The Ombudsman went back to the Council and another long wait for an answer...

*   *   *

Now to address the letter to the DLA: I wrote to the Blackpool office asking to see the letter referred to in the Council's note and I enclosed a copy of the note. When the phone rang I was surprised to hear a lady from the DLA say, "I have read your letter very carefully, would you like a copy of the whole file?" "But you can't do that, without third party approval," I said. The lady answered, "On all our note paper and letter headings we advise that we will give access to information should it be asked for. Everyone we write to has been given notice, so we can!" Amazing what forethought and efficiency, "Yes please!" It arrived quite quickly considering how many requests they had to deal with. I read it all; there was no letter from Dr. Morkane!

*   *   *

I thought about the letter from Grove Park in1991 which came in the bundle from Liverpool, it was very damning. No wonder there had been some indifferent, not to say hostile care of Andrew during his times in hospital. I took a copy and sent it to the surgeon, Mr. Rivers, who wrote it.

I said he had no right to send such a letter, I and Andrew's housemaster would have noticed if he was an alcoholic at fifteen years old! The truth was that Andrew's illness was Childhood Hereditary Pancreatitis and they were never able to control the pain. According to the text books it was typical of the disease. I also asked why it was necessary to inform the hospital in Plymouth

ANDREW'S STORY

that 'Andrew didn't get on with his father', which wasn't true. I explained as briefly as I could what had happened since the operation on Andrew and that we now know there is a 50% failure rate. We didn't blame him in any way for the failure; we all thought it was for the best at the time. Andrew had eventually agreed to the operation although he was terrified and didn't really want it done; but he needed to please his wife. He had spiralled down and there had been no help from anyone and particularly very little help from colleagues in the medical profession. Andrew was now wifeless, homeless and he was bankrupt, this as a result of not having a job and no support. He had not been told he would be disabled after the operation and it was hard for him to come to terms with that.

Surprisingly enough there was an answer from Mr. Rivers. I didn't expect it. He sympathised with the difficulties of chronic illness and the pressure it puts on families and said we know a lot more about childhood Pancreatitis now. He said it was important to know as much as possible about patients as it gave an insight into their illness and that is why clinicians should understand family relationships. I replied that whenever I wanted to understand what treatment was taking place, I was told that patient confidentiality would not allow me any information. Again he replied and I didn't expect that. He almost apologised! I left it at that... No wonder we have had such a hard time with many clinicians!

*   *   *

The local Government Ombudsman said there had been a test case and that Councils are no longer allowed to make housing benefit applications deficient. They must make a decision. The Citizens Advice Bureau opened negotiations with the Council. The Council said they thought Andrew would not be eligible and if we appealed we would not win. I returned our comment, through the CAB that if housing benefit was not granted, we would appeal, whether or not we would win. They had been as difficult as they could with me and now I would be the same with them. Shortly after that, housing benefit was granted, with three years back pay! Not a lot of good now that Andrew had lost his home and independence! No wonder Shelter say, 'Late payment causes homelessness'.

The Ombudsman said, "You have serious misgivings about the Council's assessment of medical priority, you remain of the view that you were incorrectly advised about its approach to the allocation of sheltered accommodation. The Council had admitted to the Ombudsman, they **do** have sheltered accommodation for people under sixty, in hard to let properties! (I wonder what that

ANDREW'S STORY

means!) Your continuing concerns are noted but I cannot currently determine that your position on the housing register would have been significantly better, or that you would have been offered alternative accommodation sooner had the Council dealt with your application differently. Therefore, I cannot conclude that you have been caused injustice as a result of maladministration by the Council."

After the Court case, which the Ombudsman cannot look into, Andrew had to make a fresh housing application and of this the Ombudsman said. "It is now open to you to ask for a fresh assessment of your housing need. The Council has agreed that it will refer your application to an appropriate medical adviser."

The Ombudsman said there was nothing wrong in giving a blank form to applicants to sign when requesting information from other organisations. There was nothing wrong in their dealings with the DLA. No mention of the letter to DLA from Dr. Morkane.

Housing Benefit was to be our only victory with the local council, the letter to the DLA has not been withdrawn. Andrew's DLA has been reviewed and it is still granted at the same level as before. The Ombudsman says there has been no injustice caused by their administrative fault! We still have not been told why specialist doctors were not consulted, although I have been told by an adviser, it is because the Council would have to pay for an opinion. By asking the PCT, it didn't cost anything!

We asked for Andrew to be assessed for the housing application he made after the court case, as the Ombudsman had advised. The PCT had said they would reassess and we asked for them, or a doctor who advises Government departments, to make the assessment or our new GP. Dr. Morkane now said the PCT couldn't do that as the PCT, 'didn't have the experience to do it'! Strange, they did the first time, so what happened to change matters?

He recommended a firm called Nowmedical. We did not want Nowmedical to be involved as we had heard from Shelter there were concerns over assessments from this firm. The fact that they did not work for individuals only authorities and prided themselves, according to their web site on, 'same day' assessment reports, was somewhat alarming.

The Council sent Andrew's application and statement to Nowmedical and when we received a copy of their report, we were not surprised to see it supported the Council's position. No specialists had been consulted.

ANDREW'S STORY

I wrote to Nowmedcal and asked, as they had
assessed Andrew for a condition based on an
application two years ago, would they now
reassess him for a condition three years ago? I
would pay for it. There was no reply. In all I wrote
four times including by recorded delivery, but I
never did have a reply. I asked the Council to
reassess Andrew using Nowmedical, as at the first
assessment and I would pay, but they didn't
answer either. I read on the 'net' that questions
are being asked in the 'House' about this firm.

I looked for the firm at Companies House but
could not find a company called Nowmedical at
their address.

The Local Government Ombudsman eventually
closed our case. It had taken almost four years;
they would take no more action.

A year later the Council offered Andrew a one
bedroom bungalow near us. It was an end terrace
of three with a front, side and back garden, a big
plot for him to manage, I had never seen him
gardening but the property could have been really
nice, a lot of work for a sick person though, it was
overgrown. There was a fish pond in the back
garden and fish still in it! Andrew retained an
interest in fish as marine biology had been Jane's
subject at University. Inside, the bungalow had
been partly modernised so there was a lot of work

to be done clearing up. Previously there had been a square of carpet on a concrete floor with a surround of plastic which was partly removed. It needed work on it and money to be spent! But it was a nice bungalow; I wouldn't have minded it myself! Andrew signed the tenancy contract but three weeks later had done nothing about cleaning up or moving and the first bill for rent came! Eventually he had to admit it was all too much for him to handle. He sent a letter to terminate the tenancy contract which took another month's rent, and he was very miserable. He had to pay in the region of £300 rent for a property he never moved into!

*   *   *

I tried again to find who monitors Government Guidelines, another report from another department said, "Perhaps the question was asked by phone, there is no evidence that the question was ever asked. It must go through the right procedures." So I made another request for the information by letter, this time to Yvette Cooper the Minister of Housing, no answer.

At the same time my MP sent another letter to the ODPM and his letter was sent on to the Department Of Works and Pension to be answered! What did they have to do with anything? Is somebody trying to send him on the

ANDREW'S STORY

same sort of circle that I had been sent on so many times? He wrote to the Prime Minister. I then emailed the Housing Strategy and Legislation Division for information. I kept the question free of anything personal, I had so many times been told, 'we cannot comment on personal issues'. After an exchange of nine emails including a copy of my unanswered letter to Yvette Cooper, the answer is, 'the courts effectively monitor adherence to the code of guidance'!

I emailed back, how can disabled homeless people be expected to go to court? An answer! 'I understand your son did'.

My response, *'I am not talking about a specific case, as you say you cannot comment on that. I was asking a general question, how can a disabled person, generally speaking, go to court? They may have just enough savings to preclude them from Legal Aid, that would make it impossible and they may not have anyone to advise them anyway. Court proceedings are not the first thing that pops into your mind when being made homeless! There are only twenty one days to make an appeal, after that you are out of time and can't appeal! Surely, your department should be looking at monitoring local authorities who take any opportunity to avoid their responsibilities as a way of saving money. That shouldn't be left to people who are already at a disadvantage. Is your department taking any steps to rectify the matter?'*

Their answer:

'The Department provides more than £15 million per year to help fund a number of voluntary organisations that provide assistance to homeless people. Some of these may also provide advocacy support to individuals in the event of a legal dispute, for example, Shelter and the Citizens Advice Bureaux. The help that should be available to disabled people from organisations such as the Citizens Advice Bureau and Shelter should take their disability into account.

You suggest that this Department should monitor local authorities who avoid their responsibilities. Within this Department, the Housing Strategy and Support Directorate includes a team that monitors the implementation of the Department's homelessness policies on the ground. This team includes a small group of specialist advisers who work with local authorities to encourage them to adopt innovative approaches to tackling and preventing homelessness and help them improve their service delivery. However, the Department does not have the power to intervene in individual cases where a housing applicant considers that a local authority has not fully complied with their statutory obligations towards him or her. The monitoring bodies in such a case are either the Courts or, in the case of maladministration, the Local Government Ombudsman.

The homelessness legislation does include important safeguards such as the applicant's right to ask for a review of the authority's decision on his or her application and to appeal to the county court on a point of law if dissatisfied with the review decision. Authorities are also required by law to notify applicants of these rights. But, where there is a legal dispute, only the courts have the power to review the local authority's decisions and action, and decide whether they were lawful.

More generally, strategic regulation of local authority services in England, including housing and homelessness services, is carried out by the Audit Commission. Within the Audit Commission, the Housing Inspectorate inspects and monitors the performance of a number of bodies and services including local authority housing departments'.

I asked how I could contact the monitoring 'team'. That was a step too far for them.

'In my view you have addressed your questions to the right place, namely, this Department. I am sorry if you have not received the answers that you wanted'.

Chapter 16

Help at last?

I had forgotten how far the Albert Hall is from South Kensington tube station. It was my birthday and April had bought tickets for us all to see the Cirque de Soleil. It was a dark, wet, cold and windy night, not nice to be out! Andrew found the walk difficult as he had what he called wobbly leg syndrome and he held on to my arm. Sitting was difficult because of pain and he stood up at the entrance to the auditorium when everyone was seated, but he was told to go and sit down, (Health and Safety!) He did for a while but had to get up and spent much of the time outside! Such a shame he missed much of the show and the tickets were not cheap.

He was very poorly by the end of the show and we took a taxi back to April's flat. The next day we went home on the train and he was glad to be home. Things didn't improve and sometimes he found walking very difficult, the wobbly legs wouldn't go as quick as they came! The depression didn't improve and the anti-depressant pills were changed to amatriptoline which also have some impact on pain relief.

ANDREW'S STORY

A couple of months later we went back to St.Thomas's for another procedure, which meant staying with April. On the day we were to travel home, April was flying to Edinburgh from City Airport. She had been sent to Scotland to work at Sky TV. Andrew wouldn't get up and I said come on don't mess about; we have a train to catch. He didn't speak and his behaviour was very weird. Eventually tempting him with a cup of tea and cigarette we got him up. April lives on the sixth floor and outside on her balcony, where Andrew usually went to smoke, he eyed the balcony hand rail with curiosity. Ron stayed with him while he smoked; concerned that he might try to climb over the top. We tried to reassure April that all would be well and she must leave or she would miss her flight. We said we would lock up carefully and be off as soon as we could.

We didn't worry about getting Andrew dressed as his PJ's were a bit like a leisure suit and with a coat over the top it wouldn't matter. We were getting worried that we would miss our train. We had tickets that could not be changed, if we missed that train we would have to pay for another. We got to the door but he made it plain, without speaking, that he wanted to get dressed, so to humour him and because I thought it would be quicker, we got him dressed. I thought he was going out of his mind and I just prayed that we would get home before he was sectioned.

April phoned just as we had got out of the flat to see how things were going, she was about to take off. We put on the best face we could to reassure her, the flat was securely locked, we were all OK and were off to catch the train. On the tube I said that Ron should sit down with Andrew and I would look after the cases. Suddenly Andrew got up and said, "You should be sitting down, I will stay with the cases," as normal as anything! I said I didn't think he had been well and he should sit down, did he remember how he got on the train? He could remember nothing at all! Later our GP said this was typical behaviour of a diabetic hypo, but I had never seen Andrew like that before. It was very frightening. I had only ever seen him when he had blacked out completely, this change of personality I had not witnessed before.

The diabetes was beginning to be less stable and I wondered if we were calculating the food ratios properly so I asked for an appointment with the dietician at Grove Park. Nothing happened so I phoned the department again. They said they would send an appointment, but in another month nothing came, so I phoned again! This time the receptionist made an appointment there and then, but later a dietician that we had seen before Liz, phoned to say that she wouldn't see Andrew. Why? Because he is seen in Bristol not Grove Park for diabetes and she didn't want to say anything different to what we had been told in Bristol. We haven't been told anything in Bristol. We only have the information given by the diabetic pump nurse and what we have read ourselves. Did she know the ban on Andrew had been lifted by the diabetes department now? She hedged and didn't answer.

*   *   *

I always listen to the radio when on my own working in the kitchen. There was an interesting programme on Radio 4, all about waste in the NHS. It seems that medication had gone missing from a waste disposal site. Twenty seven litres of morphine sulphate, 900kg of cocaine paste, what ever that is and eight boxes of methadone, each box containing six cartons. Hummm and Andrew was told he was a waste of NHS resources!

The PNS bulletin board that I relied on so much for contact with other people with this illness was breaking down regularly, there was so much traffic on it, I missed it greatly. When doubts were put in my mind I could ask my friends on the board if they had whatever the current problem was. There was always at least one who could advise often many more. It was always interesting to hear what other people had to say.

Eventually Stephen came to our rescue. He discussed the problem with Jim who had started the PSN web site and then he started the PSN, Pancreatitis Supporter's Network, U.K. We were back in business!

From Stephens PSN.

'Hello, I am 31 and I have AP. (Acute Pancreatitis).

I have been reading this forum for a couple of hours and to say it has made me feel better is an understatement – it's so good to actually read peoples stories and be able to relate to them. I haven't been able to speak to anyone who has suffered with AP and I have found that the most difficult thing.

My story starts last July when I had severe pain and was rushed to hospital, I was in ICU for three days after I began having breathing difficulties and I was told I nearly died which was a bit of a shock to say the least. I spent four weeks in hospital with the majority of the time being in HD. I was told it was because of gall stones and that my pancreas took a direct hit and it is now 50% dead. It was the worse time of my life but for some strange reason I thought the minute I got out of hospital things would get better, but that was when my real battle began. I couldn't eat for six weeks

ANDREW'S STORY

because I just kept being sick and I could barely get out of bed as I was so weak. I lost two stones in weight but glad to say almost a stone has popped itself back on. I was off work for four months but glad to say things are looking up for me just now, I went back to work in November and I have not had an attack for almost two weeks.

When I have an attack I honestly feel like I am dying and it is worse than labour believe me! I find it just comes on so damn quick that there is nothing that works quick enough to relieve the pain. I have oxycontin which I am going to use next time so hopefully that does the trick. I have experienced the alien thing, which is a fabulous way of describing it. One time the alien just moved in me and the pain disappeared, I also find the minute I am sick the pain just fades away, so I am generally praying damn hard for this to happen.

I think heat is a good thing and always have a hot water bottle to hand. The worst thing with AP is I feel I have a time bomb waiting to go off inside me. I just dread another attack and I get so damn stressed and depressed about it. Sometimes I wish one would just happen then I would feel I had another one to two weeks of not worrying about it happening for a while - which is a bit sick.

I am currently waiting to get my gall bladder out

and have a cyst on my pancreas drained and hopefully I will be able to go back to my carefree self.

Anyway glad I had the chance to rant about this - I feel a bit better now. Take care'

       *   *   *   **

'Welcome to the forum.

You mentioned how ranting about Pancreatitis made you feel better, that's exactly why I and many others find these forums a great help. I would never have believed that typing about my illness (I'm 28 with chronic pancreatitus for the last 7-8 years) would actually make me feel better, but it certainly does.

Just talking with other people who understand the illness is a great help.

I hope you keep on posting.

All the best'

       *   *   *

'You have my empathy. Your story is so much like my own but it was a couple of years before I discovered this forum and was then able to talk to

ANDREW'S STORY

others who knew what I was talking about. When I came to Intensive Care I was told that generally no one has an attack as bad as I had and actually survive the experience - yes it frightens the hell out of you and the mere thought of experiencing that level of pain again is also extremely frightening.

Like yourself I also had a cyst on the pancreas but the hospital was unable to drain it because the fluid within the cyst was "jelly-like." Because they could not drain it they had to operate and remove it and the part of the pancreas it was attached to. Since then my whole, or what was left of my pancreas, died. SO WHAT .... here six years later I am still alive with no pancreas my pain basically under control and Type 1 diabetes that has a mind of its own.

During those years since the first attack I have learnt a lot, much the hard way from personal experience, and much from this forum. I could have saved myself a lot of strife if I had been aware of this forum much earlier. Don't be frightened of asking questions Katrina.

Take care of yourself, take it very easy after the cyst has been drained and take great care with your diet. I assume you have read some of the postings in regards to food, diet, intake.

*Hoping you have a pain-free future in front of you.
Ray'*

        *   *   *

Social Services were again asked to make an assessment of Andrew's needs. This time by a senior Social Worker who brought with him a Community Nurse. She never said a word throughout the whole interview and we never saw her again. Pages and pages of questions were filled in.

They listed his medication which Andrew said he must rely on us to collect as there was no transport.

Oxycontin
Oxynorm
Amitriptyline
Zopiclone
Zoton
Vitamins A&D
Senna
Stemetil
Creon 40000, 25000, 10000
Humalog Insulin

Andrew said the constant vomiting meant that his teeth are decaying from acid erosion. He has now

ANDREW'S STORY

had twenty fillings and five teeth removed and a 'plate' with four false teeth on!

The assessor listed action points for Andrew to organise with his DLA. (At this time I didn't think Andrew could organise anything for anyone)

Laundry, Cleaning, Transport, Shopping, Cooking, Assistance to and from appointments.

Other action points.

Medical conditions to be dealt with by doctors
Carer support worker in contact with your parents.
Day care/ lifelong learning. Please confirm when you are well enough for this.
One to one counselling for parents.-declined.
(Later we were persuaded to undergo this, but it didn't change anything! We were offered a day of 'pampering'. I wonder why they wasted money on things like that and not practical help)?

Conclusion.

Andrew currently does not meet our criteria for help of any kind.

*   *   *

We had been out on a National Trust trip and when we got back Andrew was sitting on the floor.

I asked him what he was doing down there and he said he went to get out of bed and his legs wouldn't take his weight, he fell over. He couldn't feel them and was getting around by putting a cushion under each knee and sliding. He thought they would be better in the morning and wouldn't go to the Out of Hours Doctor. They weren't better the next day, but it was Friday. I always told him not to be ill on Friday, Saturday or Sunday as our doctor is not available on those days! After a week of this I phoned the psychiatrist as our doctor was on holiday and I wasn't sure the other GP would be sympathetic. The psychiatrist made an appointment at the Clinical Assessment Unit. I couldn't think what that was but then realised that it was the ward where A&E patients were sent until it was decided what to do with them. Andrew attended the appointment as he agreed it couldn't be left any longer, but made it clear that he was a day patient and he wasn't stopping! A full neurological examination was carried out and an MRI scan! I was impressed; people wait months for an MRI so they did take it seriously! Nothing useful was found, just a little weakness in one ankle and foot. In spite of their kind invitation to stay, there was a bed, we went home. The pain and sickness did not let up.

The next day Andrew had an appointment at our local mental health care outpatients for CBT counselling. We hired a wheelchair to get him around and later the same day he had an appointment at our own doctor's surgery. It was to remove stitches from a cut caused by a fall at home. It seems that the Councillor had phoned the doctor on duty saying that Andrew had tried to commit suicide again and was unsuccessful. He was disappointed that the councillor had shared that with the doctor; he thought he was talking in confidence. Eventually the legs got better and he could walk again.

The numbness in his legs re-occurred, but no tests could find anything wrong, although there was some weakness it eventually passed. The report said that it may or may not be organic meaning that perhaps it was all in his mind. I couldn't understand that because when they stuck pins in him, he didn't flinch and said he couldn't feel it. With the passing of time he eventually recovered from what ever it was.

From the PSN

'My husband was diagnosed with Pancreatitis about eight weeks ago. He was sent home from hospital with not much of an idea what to expect.

Saw a consultant about two weeks ago who said that he has 'grumbling Pancreatitis'. And it can go on for weeks and weeks. Since then he is much worse. The pain is so bad he can hardly walk. If he gets into a 'good position' the pain is a one out of ten. Walking the pain is one hundred. We have been told there is no treatment.

Will the pain ever go? It's been constant now since Christmas. Not a let up for even one moment.

Can anyone tell me please is this type of pain normal. Is there a diet that can help? Any advice would be appreciated. We feel alone and confused.'

Advice.

'Practicalities first: diet - low fat, high carb - no alcohol. Follow this and you are doing just about everything right for the textbook Pancreatitis diet. Of course there will be things your husband finds he cannot tolerate but that will have to be trial and error. Let me repeat - no alcohol. In any way shape or form.

There is no such thing as grumbling Pancreatitis, it's either Pancreatitis or it's not, so discount that.

Will the pain ever go – yes. But before we promise that as absolute - what sort of treatment has your husband had in hospital - presumably if they diagnosed Pancreatitis they have been

ANDREW'S STORY

treating it?

Let us know how he was treated and we'll take it from there. Don't worry - we will all help you.'

And

'...........WHERE DO YOU LIVE? If we know the country you are in we may have some idea of treatment you can expect.

You have not really given us enough information to give you any "solid and helpful" advice.

AS for the doctor saying "there is no treatment!" Unbelievable!

Let us assume your husband DOES have Pancreatitis then the first treatment should be to get the pain under control and I am afraid that generally requires a period in hospital as the first essential is to rest the pancreas and this is generally done by putting the patient in a "Nil by Mouth" situation and controlling any existing pain with pain killers.

I would like more details on your husband's condition and reaction to given situations. Does he have painkillers available???'

Joint inflammation

'These joint inflammation problems often get worse if I am building up to and during an AP attack. No one seems to know why, or of any possible link to AP but my GP thinks it must be part of what ever it is that triggers off my AP. I also have some kind of lung inflammation which no one seemed to understand but which my GP found responded well to a steroid inhaler. (After a lot of trial and error and being passed around lots of different hospital specialists).

Fortunately I have a very, very supportive GP who says he can't cure me or explain what is happening but that he will do his utmost to treat every symptom and he works to keep this promise, ranging from painkillers to physio to trying different inhalers. I wish everyone on the site had such a good GP as I really feel for people when they post about lack of support from their Doctors.

Any ideas gratefully received to see if anyone else has the same syndrome/range of symptoms as me.'

*   *   *

'Yes I have joint pain and recently some numbness in the right leg and pain at the back. I went to the GP who said all was ok probably

ANDREW'S STORY

inflammation but no cause?

*I get it in my arms too sometimes not bad and
other times like tooth ache and I have often
wondered if it was anything to do with the CP?
Maybe as most things are'*

* * *

Interesting to read your post.

*'There are signals I get which always herald a
flare-up of my Pancreatitis. I get pain in my legs
but it isn't really in the joints, it seems to be at the
insertions of tendons onto the bones. Last week I
couldn't actually put any weight on my left leg - it
was painful and kept giving way. I get swollen
joints in my fingers and knees, pain in my
shoulders, weakness in my arms and pins and
needles! There is a vein in my right wrist which
swells up. Little bruises appear on my legs.*

*I've recently had a full set of blood tests including
an autoimmune assay but haven't had the results
yet. I wonder if the cause of all this is damage to
small capillaries by circulating enzymes but
haven't found anyone who agrees with me yet!*

What a catalogue of ailments!

Anyway this is while the attack is building up then it fades away afterwards till the next time - two or three weeks later!

Best Wishes'

*   *   *

'I also get leg and arm pains and stiffness in them. I have a B12 deficiency which has stemmed from Pancreatitis. This vitamin deficiency has now caused neuropathy in my arms and legs. The latest is my knees have now gone stiff and I am some of the time having to walk with a walking stick. I wonder sometimes what next. I have a Dr. appointment on Friday so I will ask about knee stiffness.
If we all managed to get together it would be a sight for sore eyes, 😄and I guess it would be a long wait, waiting for one of us to offer to put the kettle on.'

*   *   *

'Yes I have regular blood tests for B12 deficiency, I now have the injections about every twelve weeks, but my GP gives me a blood test form to keep at home, so that if I feel that my level has dropped then I can just go for a blood test and then ring the GP the next day for the result and if necessary, go in early and get a shot. When I first

ANDREW'S STORY

started these injections I was having three a week until my level came up to the required level. This has all stemmed from my CP. Another horrible thing is that from my B12 deficiency (that had been undetected) is that I now have irreversible nerve damage peripheral neuropathy. This was all sorted out by my new GP. It happened that we moved house and this has been a god send because my GP has just floated down from heaven. If he doesn't know something that I am moaning about he will research it.

My advice is ask your GP anything and everything, and if he doesn't know hopefully he will find out for you.'

*   *   *

Andrew had been falling from time to time. On one occasion we heard the noise and found him under his book case. He tried to save himself by grabbing it but it fell on top of him. There were books everywhere and we picked him, and them up! Another time he fell on to his coffee table and Ron had to glue the leg back on. His face was quite scratched. The next day the other side of his face was cut in several places and we took him to the doctor to have this stitched up, assuming it was another nocturnal fall.

Over the next few weeks more cuts appeared on his body and the scenario of falls was becoming a little thin. The doctor thought he was doing it himself but Andrew said he had no recollection of it. He couldn't believe he would harm himself as he said, "I am in enough pain without inflicting more!"

He had been more poorly than usual when I took him to see the nurse to have more stitches out, the sickness didn't let up and he was loosing weight, I could see it! The nurse took his temperature and said it was forty; he should stop and see the doctor on duty. The doctor didn't make him wait until the end of surgery, which was good of her, but she did give him quite a lecture on self harm, he came home more depressed than ever.

The next day he was even more sleepy than usual. I had learnt how to take his blood sugar now and in the morning it was reasonable but I hadn't done it since then, so I took it again and it was twenty one! As far as I could tell he hadn't eaten anything so it should have been stable. I woke him but he couldn't seem to coordinate enough to prime the pump to give more insulin, and I didn't know how to do that! I decided I should give him an injection, something I had never done before. I made my calculation and drew up the injection and stuck it in his bottom.

ANDREW'S STORY

He didn't wake! Soon after that it occurred to me
that I didn't think he had taken any of his
medication. So I gave him some morphine tablets
as I didn't want him going into withdrawal. It was
such a job to get him to take it that I began to
wonder if this was just his normal illness! I
phoned Out of Hours and eventually a doctor rang
back and I told her the problem. She thought it
might be flu, could she speak to him? I woke him
as best I could and gave him the phone but as the
doctor spoke to him he kept dropping it. I took the
phone and said, as she was still giving him
instructions that it was me and he couldn't hold the
phone. "Do you think he needs a home visit?" "I
don't know," I said, "He is always ill." She said
she would fax a prescription to the pharmacy.
Leaving Andrew with his sister who was still
visiting from Christmas, Ron and I went to the
pharmacy. They didn't have the prescription,
although they said they thought the printing
machine was going to work, it made the noise, but
then it didn't. Phone the doctor they said but I
didn't bring the number with me. The assistant
gave me a number but it was wrong, unobtainable.
There was a buzzing, down came a shutter and
she said we are closing now, they locked up and
left!

We drove to the Out of Hours office in the hospital
and they gave us the prescription, we then drove
to another pharmacy and they filled it and closed

at once! Back home it was very difficult to get Andrew to take the pill and he couldn't drink the water without spilling most of it. I decided that we did need a home visit and phoned Out of Hours again. The recorded opening message say's if you have an emergency, replace the phone and call 999, I did.

While I was waiting for the paramedic to arrive, I took his B/G again it was 8.5, coming down nicely, but the pump was telling me it was out of insulin! The paramedic came in less than ten minutes. By now Andrew didn't respond at all. He was given oxygen and I was asked to phone for an ambulance. It also arrived in no time at all and the three men worked very hard to stabilize Andrew. He was very ill. After twenty minutes they were satisfied he could be moved and took him downstairs to the ambulance. As before, their service was faultless! I went in the ambulance with him and April followed in a car. In the ambulance I told the paramedics that I had taken Andrew to the doctor the day before and they were surprised. I then told them that Andrew had written a living will and I was wondering what to do about it. He had written it after the expert patient programme he had been on. (He never did hear about becoming a tutor for them). They asked where it was and I said on his file in hospital. "As we haven't seen it," they said, "We must treat him."

ANDREW'S STORY

My daughter and I were shown into a side waiting room in A&E, not the usual waiting room and I thought, oh he is ill! Eventually a doctor came to see us, he said it was advanced pneumonia and had we left it until the morning; it might have been too late. But he hasn't had a cold, I said and we were told, pneumonia doesn't always come from a cold. I explained about the living will and he said it was not on the file and what did we want to do about it. We decided that treatment should continue. The living will was eventually found in file four but the A&E department had file six! All the staff were as kind, helpful and sympathetic as could be, we couldn't have asked for better service. If only it had always been like that......

The next day we visited the medical assessment unit and he was sitting up. He didn't remember anything and wanted to know how he got there. We discussed with the nurse which ward he sould go into, as she said all wards can treat pneumonia. I suggested he should go to neurology because of the leg problem; he had an outpatient's appointment soon. It wouldn't be so good to send him to the diabetes ward as he is treated in Bristol. (I didn't want to say he would not be welcome there.)

We visited the next day and he was in the diabetes ward! Although far from well he was out of hospital as soon as he could stand properly, on day three! I asked social services for a discharge package but we received no help at all. At home he asked why his living will had not been followed and I explained it was in file four and they had file six. He never told me if that was good or bad and I didn't ask.

Later we were told that much of his sickness was thought to be due to scar tissue blocking the exit to his stomach, he had lost weight again. As the stomach couldn't pass food through, it rejected it in the form of vomit and this can under some circumstances contribute to pneumonia.

*   *   *

The psychiatrist said he thought Andrew's depression had worsened; he was in a 'fugue state' and so would not remember harming himself. He said that Andrew was angry inside himself over what had happened to him, he had no control over anything happening to him. This was his way of releasing his anger. He couldn't take it out on anyone else so he turned his anger in on himself; it must all be his own fault, he had been told that enough times! In spite of the psychiatrist seeing him each week, the cuts were getting longer and deeper and more often. The crisis team were called in and I was relieved to have the help I believe we should have had five

ANDREW'S STORY

years ago. Why don't people listen? This was not the first crisis we had to get him through without any help. I now believe there have been at least three attempted suicides. The pain clinic psychiatrist said it was just a cry for help, but there wasn't any, just blame from her. Eventually Andrew was asked to go into the local mental health hospital. He said, "Give me a bit longer to see if it stops," he didn't want to be in any hospital, especially not the 'nuthouse' as he called it, but it didn't stop. He was given an ultimatum, come in as a voluntary patient or we will use the mental health act and section you for your own safety.

At first we never found what he had been using as a weapon against himself, although we all searched his flat. At his request we took away anything sharp. As time went on we found a hacksaw left out for us to find in the workshop. We showed it to Andrew, he shuddered and turned away, "How could I?" He said. I began to wonder if he could be sleep walking. There had been episodes of this before. The compassion our GP showed, as he stitched him up again and again was remarkable and we will be forever grateful. Andrew went to the surgery expecting to be 'told off' but he wasn't! As the doctor said to me, he is a very disturbed young man. Who wouldn't be?

Andrew was to be admitted to hospital the following Friday and through the week there were many discussions and soul searching on whether or not he was a 'nut'. We explored the fact that one in four of the population would have some sort mental health issue during their life time and it was nothing to do with whether or not you are 'nuts'. While he and others thought of hospitals as nuthouses there would be little understanding of the issues involved, or his own difficulties. I think he was really asking for my understanding that he was not mad and the abusive terms being used were to probe my feelings on the subject. He needed the support of knowing that we wouldn't abandon him.

It is obvious to me that Andrew's physical and mental health are very fragile now, so why the big divide between the two disciplines? As one feeds the other, should the two disciplines be so far apart?

So much for the clever, intelligent people who assessed him as 'able to live on the streets without detriment the same as any other homeless person'! Where are they now? Do they ever have to go into a loved one's bedroom and find them covered with blood? Will they ever be brought to book for what they have done?

ANDREW'S STORY

The bed for Friday didn't materialise and Monday
was the next target day, but that too passed by. I
began to think if they don't hurry up he will change
his mind and they will not get him into hospital
without a struggle. He said he was better as there
had been no 'problem' for a week! He didn't need
to go; I didn't comment one way or the other
fearing that whatever I said would make things
worse. With all the money being poured into
health care why isn't there a bed for someone in
crisis?

A week later a bed was available and a very meek
and mild, and very frightened young man was
admitted to the psychiatric hospital for
assessment. His medication was taken off him
but he was assured that he could access it though
a nurse anytime he needed it. He had a sore eye
and they said they would get the doctor to look at
it, his immunity system seems shot to pieces
these days. We visited on Saturday and he said
he had watched the rugby that afternoon.
Watching the TV is ruled by majority he said. I
asked how he had seen rugby then and he said a
nurse wanted to see it and they don't argue with
him, he is six foot tall and an ex-rugby player!

He had found where to help himself to tea, it was
on tap all day which was good as he never
stopped drinking, he always had a dry mouth and
was always thirsty. I asked if he had eaten

anything, "I had a doughnut at supper (9pm) last night." No dinner? No. He said that people 'kick off' in here and when the alarm bell rings they have to go back to their rooms and stay there. I asked if anyone had been to see him, "No its weekend, what a funny time to take someone into hospital." He wanted to come home for the day on Sunday and staff said that was OK. When we got to the hospital, the outside door was locked and we couldn't just walk in as we had before. We were told someone had been playing up, 'it is a pity as everyone suffers then,' said the receptionist as he let us in.

We found Andrew in his room, his eye was weeping constantly, it was very sore and had red 'fingers' running from it down his cheek. "What did the doctor say?" I asked and he said, "I haven't seen one!" I took him to Out of Hours and we got some eye drops for it. To my surprise he went back to the hospital like a lamb. I think he accepted that he did need help.

On Monday we visited and he was still asleep at 3.30pm. Nothing unusual about that but how could they assess him? I woke him and his eye was stuck together. I stopped a passing nurse and asked if she would bring something to bathe his eye. "I can't touch it," she said, "The doctor hasn't seen it." I assured her that a doctor had seen it, as I had take him to Out of Hours

ANDREW'S STORY

yesterday. "He has to be seen by our doctor before I can touch it." I asked for some cotton wool, I would do it myself. She didn't know if there was any and had to ask someone else who found it in their treatment room. I bathed his eye which was well stuck up, it was still weeping badly and put some drops in it.

I looked at the record book for his blood sugar and it had not been taken all day. He pulled the cord for a nurse to ask for medication, he hadn't had any yet. I said shall we do your B/G and as I picked up the monitor, the nurse walked in. You can come down to the treatment room to do that if you like, while I get his medication. As we got into the room the alarm went off and he rushed off telling another nurse to see to Andrew's medication. She was about to unlock the cabinet when she turned to me and said rather aggressively, "Will you wait outside?" As I walked out I said I would wait outside, that was no problem to me, but she should know that I was invited in, I hadn't pushed my way in uninvited. When she came out she said she was sorry but didn't know who I was, she had just come back from a week's leave and she hadn't met Andrew before either.

I explained that Andrew's B/G should be taken four to six, or even eight times a day and it hadn't been done at all so far today. Why hadn't he done it himself, she asked. He was asleep and no one woke him up! Then I asked who his named nurse is? She went off to look at the list and came back saying, she was on nights last week and is on annual leave this week. That would be why we haven't seen her then!

In his room Andrew said he didn't go out of the room now as he was frightened and he began to weep. I asked what he had eaten in the last four days and he said, "A doughnut." "Do you want to go home?" "Yes!" He said. "OK let's go home!" I called the nurse and said can we have Andrew's medication, we are leaving. The head nurse arrived and wanted to know what was going on and why did we want to take him home.

I asked if he knew that Andrew had not eaten anything since he had been there. No, he didn't know there was a food problem; I said he found it difficult to keep anything down and hadn't eaten, he wasn't anorexic, he has a mal-absorption problem. Did he know his named nurse was on leave? No, I will check that! I said the doctor had not come to see his eye, (which was still weeping badly and looked very sore). While it was understandable that no one had come to see him over the weekend, he had been there four days and had seen no one, how could they assess him, he was only there for a week? The nurse said there had been difficult patients in the unit just

ANDREW'S STORY

now and they had to be dealt with. They spoil it
for everyone. I said I thought they would expect
that in a place like this. Did he know that Andrew
was frightened to go out of his room now? He
opened his mouth but closed it again and then
said, "We are short staffed and we have let
Andrew down. He has not had the service he is
entitled to receive. I would love to work with him,
one to one, but it hasn't happened I'm sorry. I'll
get his medication, but you must see the doctor
before you leave." We waited fifty minutes and a
doctor came, he wanted to know why we were
taking him home and I went through it again and
then asked, what would you do if it were a child of
yours? The same as you I expect, he said!

The next day I had to go back for the insulin, it's
kept separately in a fridge and we went home
without it. I was greeted warmly enough and the
nurse in charge said he had spoken to the
consultant and would Andrew go to the hostel
which had been talked about previously, next
Friday? I said I would ask him and I also said how
we appreciated the continuing care, I had
expected to be back on my own with this problem,
as I had been for the last five years. "No we
wouldn't do that; I hope Burton's Orchard will work
out for Andrew." I really felt he meant it. Thank
you!

Andrew was to go for a two week assessment and he agreed to one week but stayed for two in the end. The atmosphere in Burton's Orchard was completely different, calm and peaceful and with, mostly, caring staff! It is a place for recovering mental health patients to stay as a sort of halfway house, trying to prepare them for the 'outside world'. It was so close to town Andrew could walk in and shop, always a priority with him! He now had a team of six looking after him. A consultant, his senior house officer, an occupational therapist from the crisis team, a social worker, the manager of Burton's Orchard and Sue, whoever she was! After all these years of no one, now there were six! There was to be a meeting of the professionals and we were invited. But the meeting started without us! Andrew had asked that we be there. Almost two hours later he was asked in and they said we would be asked in, in a moment, they wanted to talk to Andrew first on his own.

By then I was pretty upset, did they think I had nothing better to do than sit around for two hours doing nothing? We were invited in at last to be told what they had decided! As Andrew was so much better than when he was at home with us, they had asked him to stay for a month to see how it all went! Were they implying it was being at home with us that was the problem? I felt I had to say that Andrew was at home with us as no one

ANDREW'S STORY

else had offered help when he was made homeless. The consultant, a kindly man really, said, "We must put the past behind us and look to the future." But the past shapes our future, and I knew something they didn't, but I couldn't break Andrew's trust! It was still happening. Eventually he told them.

We were asked if we had anything to say. "Yes," I answered, as we know Andrew best, I thought we were to be part of the meeting, not brought in at the end to hear what the experts had decided. As we had all been there for two hours and it was 4.30 pm, I didn't think they would want to stay for another two hours and re-run the whole meeting, I had better not say anything. If Andrew wanted to stay at Burton's Orchard, that was fine by us, we were happy if that was considered best for him, it wasn't a case that we wouldn't or couldn't let go! I felt that is what they were implying.

During the previous week I had phoned to speak to the OT on four occasions but he was never there and never returned my calls. Eventually he said, "I had to get Andrew's permission before I could speak to you." I told him that was all he had to say to me, he should not have simply ignored my calls!

He suggested that Andrew should rent a private flat and live independently from us! We had been there twice before and it didn't work! I said I would need to know what support would be available. What is his diagnosis? What did they think was wrong with him? 'That's what we are assessing him for now.' After five years! The OT said that we might like to stand guarantor for the rent. If that's what they think best, they can sort it out! I'm too worn to go down that road again. But I think Andrew has gone, he won't be back other than to visit, maybe.....until the next crisis that is. Just a bit of help at the right time might have saved all this agony. When will they ever learn?

Four months after treatment began at Burton's Orchard, there has been little progress. The weekly psychiatric sessions have not taken place. The occupational therapist has not been back to take Andrew to any other outside organisations and little happens at Burton's Orchard. There has been one 'outing' for residents but there has been no art therapy, reading groups, gardening, cooking or anything.
There is no requirement for residents to help with household chores and no cleaner, so the 'support staff' cook and clean when they should be doing other duties.

There has been no progress in independent living, it's difficult if not impossible to contact the doctors and difficult to contact the manager, they all seem

ANDREW'S STORY

to be at 'meetings'. The rest of the team of six have never been seen again.

I will continue to fight for a fair deal for Andrew and all those who are let down by the system, I cannot and will not stop, however unpopular it makes me. Things have got to change.

Burton's Orchard is to close and the facility transferred to a town fourteen miles away. What good is that to the people here? After all the changes in the health system, mental health is still a Cinderella service and one in four of us may need mental health care during our lives.

*   *   *

We have tried to get justice for Andrew from a council housing department who say Andrew is not medically vulnerable, we have failed.

We have tried to obtain a copy of the council's policy for assessing medical vulnerability and they do not answer letters or phone calls.

We have tried to find out what is medical vulnerability from the PCT and the council and failed.

We have tried to find out why it is OK for him to live on the streets when he is so ill, and failed.

We have tried to find who is responsible for the crisis and to extract an apology from them, and failed.

All this because a doctor couldn't fill in two tick boxes properly!

Of the 19,000 complaints to the Local Government Ombudsman last year, some were resolved locally but he upheld fewer than 100!

None of the authorities involved will take any responsibility, the complexity of the situation doesn't mean they understand the problems in a human way, it means they have the opportunity to push issues round in circles and they do this at every opportunity.

Authority should be there to help, that's what they are paid for, but it isn't.

One third of under seventeen year olds with ASBO orders have mental health issues according to Mind. One in four adults will have mental health issues at some point in their lives.

It seems balancing the books is important than people. All Andrew needed was sheltered accommodation and a little support. It was too much to ask.

ANDREW'S STORY

From Andrew, the first interest in doing anything creative in many years, perhaps there is hope:

Too many secrets and too many lies

Too many unforgotten memories and many muffled cries.

Too many words I wish I had never said

Too many nights of fear, anxiety and dread.

Far easier to pretend and be okay

Far easier to let things slip away.

Easier, yes, why shouldn't it be?

But do I really know you?

Do you know me?

Far easier to hide in the dark, far away

Safe from reality, safe from the problem that won't go away.

I could scream, I could shout,

People might look and people might stare,

But ask yourself this,

Would anyone really care?

Footnote.

After Andrew left his two roomed flat we were asked to pay Council tax on both our house and on his two rooms even though he did not live there any more.

In order to have the tax put back to one account as it had been for 30 years, we had to spend yet more of our retirement fund to have the rooms put back as they were. We had to take the kitchen out, the plumbing removed and the wiring put back as it was. We put our house on the market,   I just couldn't face all that!

ANDREW'S STORY

Appendix 1

From
Healthcare Commission

08 February 2005

Dear Richard,

Re: Notification to delay in review process

I am writing to update you on my progress with your case.

I am sorry to have to advise you that I am still not in a position to carry out my initial review. The reason for this delay is that I am trying to obtain a copy of the judgement of the court hearing back in March 2004. I understand that the PCT's process for assessing medical vulnerability was considered at the hearing and therefore I need to see what was said.

I can assure you that I will keep you informed of the situation and I thank you for your patience during my enquiries.

Please accept my apologies for this and I hope the delay has not caused you or Richard undue concern or inconvenience.

Brenda Prentice

Yours sincerely

Ms. Wray
Case Manager

(I wondered who Richard was)!

ANDREW'S STORY

From the Healthcare Commission

March 2005

Dear Andrew,

Re: Decision from the initial review of your complaint.

This letter is to advise you of the outcome of the initial review of your complaint. The case file and the documents you provided have been fully considered. A manager has also reviewed my decision.

I have already explained to you that I am unable to consider the decision made in respect of Andrew's housing application, which was made by the Borough Council. I can only consider the process by which a medical opinion was provided by the PCT.

Your complaint has raised three issues and I shall deal with each one in turn;

1. **The process by which Taunton Deane PCT, through the Directory of Public Health, provided a medical opinion to the local authority's housing department in relation to an assessment of medical vulnerability.**

I have decided to ask Taunton Deane PCT to take further action about this aspect of your complaint because the assessment request form that GPs are asked to complete is too restrictive.

Under the Housing Act 1996, local councils only have to ensure housing is available if they consider the applicant to be vulnerable. Local councils are required to seek and consider medical and social advice as to an applicant's vulnerability but the final decision on the question of vulnerability rests with the local council.

The definition of vulnerability is not a precise one and is open to interpretation. In addition, there is no recognised process by which councils should seek medical opinion and each council or authority makes it own arrangements. Some employ a doctor to assess applications while others rely on the views of the applicant's GP.
The process used by your Borough Council has been in place for a number of years, firstly through the old Somerset Health Authority and latterly through the Public Health Directorate of the PCT. An assessment request is made to the person's GP, via the Director of Public Health at the PCT. The process has remained virtually unchanged, other than the small change in the wording of the vulnerability criteria as explained in the PCT's letter to you date August 5th 2004 and a letter of

guidance sent to all GP practices on December 6th 2004. A copy of which is enclosed for your information.

The process by which a medical opinion is provided was clearly explained in the PCT's letter dated August 5th 2004. A copy of the form that the PCT sends to a GP asking for their views was enclosed with the letter.

Having considered the process and spoken to one of the Healthcare Commission's GP advisers, I am concerned that the form used by the PCT is too restrictive as it only asks for details of conditions that interfere with mobility and mental health problems. I have sought advice from the Office of the Deputy Prime Minister, which is responsible for the legislation regarding homelessness. Their advice is that physical disabilities or long term acute illnesses, such as those defined by the Disability Discrimination Act 1995, should also be considered.

I have recommended that the PCT review the form, in conjunction with the Borough Council if necessary, to ensure that the GP also considers any medical problems which might make a person vulnerable. I have also suggested that they provide an area on the form for GPs to make comments, rather than expecting them to write a separate letter. I have asked that they send a copy of the revised form to you for your information and a copy to me for my file.

Whilst I appreciate that this is too late to help your son, Andrew, I hope that the changes I have recommended will ensure that when the local authority is considering applications in the future, it will be able to make a fully informed decision.

If you are still dissatisfied after further local action has been taken by PCT, you can then ask the Healthcare Commission to look again at your complaint.

2. **The PCT was aware of the reputation and standard of service of the GP practice that Andrew was registered with at the time and therefore should not have provided an opinion based on advice received from that GP.**

I have decided to take no further action on this issue because from the information provided to me, I am satisfied that at the time of Andrew's application the performance of the practice in question was not giving the PCT cause for concern. They sought the opinion of Andrew's GP in accordance with their procedure for providing a medical opinion.

ANDREW'S STORY

The PCT has procedure for the identification and support of doctors whose performance is giving cause for concern and this was in place at the time of Andrew's application.

The procedure clearly identifies the types of information which may highlight poor performance and these include complaints, PALS contacts and a number of practice indicators, which the PCT routinely monitors through its Clinical Governance Directorate. Each practice has a clinical governance review file in which such information is held. Staff throughout the PCT know that information for inclusion in the file must be sent to the Clinical Governance Department. Indeed, the concerns that you expressed were passed on to that department in accordance with the process. These files are confidential and are formally reviewed on a regular basis. If during the review there appears to be cause for concern, the poor performance procedure is started.

3.   **The PCT ignored numerous requests by you for information.**

I have decided to take no further action on this issue because the PCT's complaints file shows that they responded to requests for information made by you as appropriate. Unfortunately, a number of your requests were related to confidential information, which was not in the public domain and which the PCT was not in a position to make available to you under the Data Protection Act 1990. Linda's letter of September 10th 2004 explained that this was the case. However, it would have been more helpful if they had made you aware of this at an earlier opportunity.

The PCT's response dated August 5th 2004 apologised for the fact that your letter of May 25th 2004 was not acknowledged and that staff had been reminded of the need to respond promptly.

I can appreciate that the fact I am taking no further action may be disappointing news for you, however I can assure you that I have given careful consideration to all the available evidence before reaching this decision.

If you are dissatisfied with this decision you can appeal to the Health Service Ombudsman. For further details about how you can contact the Ombudsman, please find enclosed an information sheet called 'Useful Contacts'. You may want to contact your local Independent Complaints Advisory Service (ICAS) to assist you. Their details can also be found on the information sheet.

If you have any questions about any aspect of this letter, please do not hesitate to contact me.

Yours sincerely,

Ms. Wray
Case Manager

Brenda Prentice

From Director of Public Health.

To All Practice Managers   **6th**
December

2004

Re: Vulnerable Single People and Homelessness

I am aware that general practitioners frequently receive requests from local authority housing officers, usually via a letter from me, for an opinion about a patient's 'vulnerability' in relation to the Housing Act 1996. My purpose in writing therefore is to assist general practitioners to respond in a manner that best serves the patient in terms of their health and welfare.

Under the Housing Act 1996, local councils only have to ensure housing is available if they consider the applicant to be vulnerable. Vulnerability is therefore of fundamental importance in terms of a homeless person's ability to access housing. Regrettably, the definition of vulnerability is open to interpretation and not applied consistently by all housing officers, with the result that some people who are extremely vulnerable don't receive the help that the law aims to provide.

ANDREW'S STORY

The accepted definition is that if a person were to become homeless, their health and difficulties would make them less able to fend for themselves so that injury or detriment will result, where a less vulnerable person would be able to cope without harmful effects (Courts of Appeal, ex-parte Pereira, 1999). When you are contacted by local councils to comment on whether someone is vulnerable, it would be most helpful if your comments took account of the above.

The legislation clearly places the responsibility for such decisions with local councils. However, they are required to seek a medical opinion from an appropriate source, and any comments you make will have a strong influence on the decision.

I feel therefore it's important that you are aware of the legal definition of vulnerability in terms of housing assistance and I would ask that you keep this letter for reference in future requests from local councils.

Should you require further information or wish to discuss these or any related matters, please contact me.

Dr. Morkane
Director of Public Health

Brenda Prentice

From

Healthcare Commission (again).
29 March 2005

Dear Andrew,

Re: Independent review of your complaint.

Thank you for your letter of 25 March 2005 and the enclosures and also for your phone call of that date.

I enclose a copy of the judgement. I am sorry I didn't realise you wanted it returning otherwise it would have been sent back to you sooner.

As I explained in my letter of 22 March 2005, the PCT have been asked to review the form in question. Once they have done this, and if you remain dissatisfied, you do have the right to ask the Healthcare Commission to look again at this aspect of your complaint only. The second review would involve a different case manager in looking at this aspect of your complaint and the action taken by the PCT to resolve it. Again, they would not be able to review the opinion made in respect of Andrew but only at the process.

Issues two and three have been reviewed and as no further action is to be taken, you can ask the

ANDREW'S STORY

Ombudsman to look at these two issues now. I enclose a leaflet explaining the role of the Ombudsman. Inside are details of their Helpline and I am sure they can advise you what aspects the Ombudsman can consider.

In respect of the comments made in your letter, I shall address them in turn;

1. The requirement for local councils to seek and consider medical and social opinion is clearly set out in the Housing Act 1996. In addition, in 2002 a Homelessness Code of Guidance was issued to Local Authorities. Section 8.15 reinforces the need for medical opinion and I enclose a copy of the relevant section. Further information and the full document is available in homelessness section of the website of the Office of the Deputy Prime Minister at www.odpm.gov.uk.

    I am afraid that I am unable to comment on why the PCT has not changed the form earlier.

2. The role of clinical governance is one recognised across the NHS and the principles have been in place for years. In my experience of primary care trusts it is usual for issues such as those you have

raised to be passed on to the clinical governance section so they can be held in one place and collated to give as wider a picture as possible of a practice or practitioner. I do not know if feedback from the Community Health Council was fed into clinical governance but I would expect so. At the time of Andrew's application PALS would indeed have been in its infancy but today it is an established service and a rich area for feedback for NHS organisations. As I explained to you on the phone, my review concentrated on the PCT at the time of Andrew's request and at the time of your complaint and I am not in a position to comment on what is happening now.

The number of complaints received against the Practice was provided in confidence and unfortunately I am not able to disclose this.

With respect to the opinion given by Andrew's GP, he responded to the questions asked of him on the form, which I have already indicated I feel are too narrow. Further to your intervention, this opinion was reviewed.

3.   The PCT has made available a Publication Scheme according to the Freedom of

ANDREW'S STORY

Information Act 2002. It is available on
their website and I enclose a copy for your
information. This sets out what information
is available and how to apply. I hope that it
is of assistance to you.

As I explained in my letter of 22 March
2005, my decision to take no further action
is based on the requests for information
you have made and the PCT's responses
to those requests.

With regard to the information used for my report,
some of the information was provided by the PCT
in confidence, however much of it was
communication between you and the PCT and
other information, such as policies and
procedures, which should be available through the
publication scheme. Regarding my contact with
the Office of the Deputy Prime Minister, this was
done by phone. They referred me to the guidance
I mentioned earlier in my letter and once I had
read the guidance, we had a discussion about
vulnerability and about the form that Taunton
Deane PCT were using. I have already indicated
that they were concerned at the wording of the two
questions and they referred to section 8.17 and
suggested that this should be indicated on the
PCT's form.

I hope that this has clarified the situation for you.

Brenda Prentice

Yours sincerely

Ms. Wray
Case Manager

ANDREW'S STORY

March 2005

To Taunton Deane Primary Care Trust

Dear Primary Care Trust,

Healthcare Commission Report

I have received the report from the Healthcare Commission along with a copy of your letter 6th Dec. to Practice Managers in the area. I look forward to receiving a copy of the revised form when it is available.

I wonder if you wish to add or make any other comment to the advice given to the housing department before I consider whether to approach the Health Ombudsman?

I am happy to make time to discuss anything with you or your team members to try and find a way forward.

We would also be able to discuss why the GP so badly misjudged the situation. His unhelpful referral letter to the Royal Liverpool Hospital wasted everyone's resources. It did not take into account that when Andrew walked to the surgery, he did so by selecting points of rest on the way, such as low walls, seats en route and so on. Also on many occasions I drove him to the surgery.

The GP also seems to have forgotten that Andrew is prescribed opiates as he is a very sick young man and not for recreational purposes.

Any standard medical text book tells how difficult this condition is to deal with. Certainly an enquiry of Andrew's specialists would have confirmed that.

A request for hospital notes from a Liverpool hospital was ignored until a solicitor's letter prompted these to be returned, that cost £75. We found there was a letter sent to the GP after the appointment but Andrew was never informed of this and it was never discussed with him.

Yours sincerely

ANDREW'S STORY

**From the Council file obtained by the
Information Officer.**

1st. March 2004
PALS Officer
Taunton Deane Primary Care Trust
Taunton

Dear Madam,

I am writing regarding the meeting held on
Tuesday 24th February 2004.

I have a number of concerns regarding the way
the meeting was handled and would like to draw
them to your attention. The Council's Allocations
manager who was at the meeting was also
present at the meeting shares these concerns.

Firstly I would like to point out that the attendance
of Mrs Ather and myself at this meeting was purely
voluntary. As you are aware a decision regarding
Andrew's homeless application has already been
made and the application has also been subject to
statutory review. The matter will shortly be
proceeding to Court. My understanding when
invited to attend was that the purpose of the
meeting was to discuss Andrew's present situation
amongst the attending agencies.

What actually happened in my opinion was that considerable pressure was placed upon one Authority (Taunton Deane Housing Services) to reverse a statutory decision that had been taken and that the majority of the other agencies present used their influence to add to that pressure.

I am fully aware from experience that meetings such as these can be difficult to handle, however I do believe that this meeting was chaired unprofessionally. Again my understanding was that the Chair's role was to 'control' the meeting, making sure that each Agency was given opportunity to speak whilst as Chair remaining as neutral as possible. In my opinion from the very outset an 'anti Council' stance was adopted by yourself that ran through the entire meeting.

Before the meeting you whispered to me that there was a problem. However, rather than taking me to one side and explaining what the problem was, thus giving me the opportunity to address the matter in my mind, you merely told me that it would become clear as we proceeded.
I was then surprised and disappointed by your opening remark to myself when you asked me to explain to those present what had gone wrong with Andrew's application. Immediately I was put on the back foot and the impression was given to the other attending agencies that the Council was guilty of making a mistake when dealing with the

homeless and housing applications. I do not need to point out to you that just because the Council makes a decision that an individual applicant is dissatisfied with, that it can then be assumed that an error has been made with the processing of that application.

My disappointment was compounded further a little later on in proceedings when I was attempting to answer a query from Andrew's mother as to why the Council had not sought medical guidance on Andrew's condition when he first made a housing application to us. My explanation was rudely interrupted by laughter from yourself. When I asked for an explanation none was forthcoming and whilst your laughter may have not been connected to what I was saying, because you did not explain the cause of it I believe that the other agencies would have interpreted your laughter as being a sarcastic response to the Council taking what you believed to be an unreasonable stance on this particular matter.

Throughout the meeting reference was made to a standard letter that had been sent from the Health Protection Unit to the General Practitioner. On numerous occasions I indicated that in light of concerns that you had raised regarding its contents I would take the matter up with the PCT prior to them taking over the management of these processes from the HPA. Despite me saying this you persisted in pursuing this point until my colleague felt it necessary to interrupt and reinforce the point that I had previously made.

I am sorry that I have had to write to you in this manner but I feel very strongly about the way this meeting was handled. I look forward to your comments and hope that any further meetings that are called about Andrew or any other housing applicant are managed more effectively.

Yours sincerely

Mr. Jones

Homeless and Advice Manager (According to the PCT and the housing department, this letter was never addressed or answered)

ANDREW'S STORY

From Healthcare Commission   18th May 2006

Dear Andrew,

Further to your letter of April 17th 2006, I have now had the opportunity to discuss the contents with Ms Wray.

Your request for copies of the information provided by the PCT is being processed in accordance with the freedom of Information Act and copies will follow in due course.

I have been advised by Ms. Wray that despite her letter of November 2nd. 2004 advising you that she was going to request a copy of Andrew's medical records from the PCT, the medical records were not requested. The reason for this was because her review looked at how the information was provided to the local council by the PCT and as the PCT did not have sight of Andrew's records, it was not necessary for Ms. Wray to do so. Ms. Wray thought that this had been explained to you at the time and apologised if this was not the case.

In response to your question as to what Ms. Wray took into account when considering the court judgement, Ms. Wray has told me that the PCT informed her that their process for assessing medical vulnerability was considered by the court and that it was deemed to be appropriate. Ms. Wray was not prepared to take them at their word but wished to see for herself what was said and this is why she wanted to see a copy of the judgement. Ms. Wray has advised me that she noted that the judge was satisfied with the process but she did not take the judge's ruling into account as this concerned the actions of the local council and was therefore outside her review.

I hope this further explanation is helpful.

Yours sincerely,

James Johnstone

Senior Complaints and Policy Manager.

(Actually what the judge said was 'signally irrelevant questions were asked')

ANDREW'S STORY

From the Taunton Deane PCT To Healthcare Commission

5 August 2005

Dear Ms Wray

Independent review

I refer to your letter of 9 August 2005 regarding the independent review of the complaint.

I acknowledge that it has taken some time to review the procedure relating to medical assessment for housing applications. You will appreciate that this progress involves the Local Authority as well as the Primary Care Trust and therefore the timescale for the review has not been wholly within the Trust's control. I nevertheless accept that the delay has been regrettable and apologise for this shortcoming.

I understand that Dr Morkane, Director of Public Health, has spoken to you about the form and trust that this conversation clarified the issues in relation to correspondence used to assess medical vulnerability for housing.

As you discussed with Dr Morkane, procedures for dealing with medical assessment for housing applications vary significantly between Primary

Care Trusts and Local Authorities, as do the questions asked to ascertain medical conditions and vulnerability.

The letter used by Taunton Deane Primary Care Trust sent to general practitioners in Dr Morkane's name, has been in place for several years, and was initiated under the former Somerset Health Authority. This letter is similar to that used by other Primary Care Trusts in Somerset, though not all.

The Taunton Deane Primary Care Trust letter was modified last year, following discussions with the Housing Department at Taunton Deane Borough Council arising from the complaint. The letter has now been further modified, and I enclose a copy of the revised format. I confirm that the amendments reflect comments made by Shelter.

I have, as requested, copied this letter to Andrew's mother, but would emphasise that this letter only applies to people covered by the homeless legislation. As you know Andrew is not homeless, but he is on the housing list at Taunton Deane Borough Council.

I can confirm, however, that the Primary Care Trust remains willing to review Andrew's priority points on the housing list should we be asked to

ANDREW'S STORY

do so by the Housing Department at Taunton Deane Borough Council.

I hope that this response addresses the issues you raised and again apologise that this process has taken longer than the Primary Care Trust would have wished.

Yours sincerely

Edward Colgan
Chief Executive

Brenda Prentice

July 2006

To

Director of Corporate Development and Human Resources
Taunton Deane Primary Care Trust

Dear Mr. Brice,

Thank you for replying on behalf of your complaints manager. Her Personal Assistant could have made a reply in a timely fashion; this is the 4th or 5th time I have had to remind your staff about acknowledgements of correspondence, in spite of your 'Memo'.

I understand that you think the matter of Mr. Jones' letter has been dealt with in the files the PCT has sent to the Healthcare Commission. I could not see this letter in the copy of the file they sent me. So, again I ask for a copy of the PCT's reply to Mr. Jones letter at the borough council.

In your letter of the 12th June you say at 9. (your numbering) you act as a link between the Council and the GP. If that is the case why didn't the Council go straight to the GP? It is the PCT who supplied the information which was incorrect. That was the PCT's responsibility. When will that be acknowledged?

ANDREW'S STORY

The question of why Dr. Morkane says he now does not have the practical experience of reviewing…etc. is not answered. Previously the PCT was happy to supply this information. What has changed? Your Chief Executive says they will be happy to reassess Andrew's need and now says they can't, you don't have the expertise, ask NowMedical?
What changed?

You are wrong to say Andrew's application had a judicial review, it did not, who told you it did?

What the judge said was, where expert advice is obtained, it must be reliable. He also said that someone else might have taken a more sympathetic line; the Council were within their right to find the way they did. He did not go into the question of, whether the information given by the PCT was correct. I ask you again, if five major health problems do not make someone medically vulnerable, what does?

Please don't hide behind the Healthcare Investigation; if there is nothing to be concerned about, there is nothing to fear in answering properly.

Yours sincerely,

Brenda Prentice

09 August 2005

From Healthcare Commission To Taunton Deane PCT

Dear Mr Colgan

Re: Independent review

I wrote to you on March 22nd 2005 outlining the decision of my review of the complaint. In my letter I asked the PCT to take further action and review the form used to provide a medical opinion.

It is now over four months since I returned the matter to the PCT and neither the complainant nor I have received any further information from you. I contacted Linda Pope, Corporate Development and Complaints Manager, last month for an update and she explained that the PCT was still consulting with the local authority on this matter and that the discussions had widened to include future provision of this service.

I am concerned that this matter is dragging on and that in the meantime assessments are being undertaken using the old form. I therefore recommend that the PCT update the form as I requested now as an interim measure to cover any assessments that arise before the wider review is completed. Please take account of any recommendations made by Shelter when redesigning the form.

The form should be redesigned within the next 20 working days and a copy sent to the complainant and one to me for my file.

I am copying this letter to the Strategic Health Authority for them to monitor the progress of the review of the provision of this service in the future.

I look forward to hearing from you.

Yours sincerely,

Ms. Wray
Case Manager

Brenda Prentice

September 2005

From

**Dorset and Somerset
Strategic Health Authority**

Dear Andrew,

Thank you for your letter of the 22nd September concerning Taunton Deane Primary Care Trust.

You will by now have received a response to your earlier letter of the 20th September in which I explain that this Strategic Health Authority does not have responsibility for investigating complaints against the Primary Care Trust and that I am unable to comment on this matter.

Yours sincerely

Sir Ian Caruthers

Chief Executive.

ANDREW'S STORY

To Strategic Health Authority

29th September 2005

Dear Sir Ian,

Thank you for your letter of the 22nd. September 05

I am aware that the Strategic Health Authority does not have responsibility for investigating complaints.

According to its web site, it does include the following:

"Through establishing robust performance management arrangements, holding to account and supporting Primary Care Trusts, NHS Trusts, clinical networks and the Dorset and Somerset Workforce Development Confederation to deliver their local priorities and improved services outlined in 'The NHS Plan' and National Service Frameworks, including the NHS Cancer Plan."

I assumed, like Ms. Wray, that you would want to know how the Taunton PCT deals with letters like the one I sent you a copy of. The PCT doesn't answer them! They should be 'held to account.'

Brenda Prentice

Please tell me, what does qualify as medically vulnerable? This is a general question to which there should be a general answer.

This is not referring specifically to my son who, as you know, has five major health conditions.

Yours sincerely,

ANDREW'S STORY

From Parliamentary and Health Service Ombudsman

20 June 2006

Dear Andrew,

Further to our telephone conversation on 19 May and your subsequent email and postal correspondence, I can now update you on progress with the investigation of your complaints.

You complain on behalf of your son about Taunton and Deane PCT (the PCT) and the Healthcare Commission. During our telephone conversation we agreed that there were six key parts to your complaint that could be investigated by the Health Service Ombudsman:

1) Taunton Deane PCT gave inaccurate information about the medical vulnerability to the local housing authority, resulting in lack of appropriate housing allocation for your son.

[You have told me that the PCT was aware that the medical vulnerability housing assessment form was inadequate a year before the assessment of your son. You also complain that the PCT's assessment of medical vulnerability was based simply on the GP's completion of two tick boxes on this form and the PCT did not review the medical records or seek expert opinion from the Specialist treating him.]

2) The Healthcare Commission asked the PCT to amend the form used to assess medical vulnerability in association with Shelter, but Shelter say that they were not consulted and still have concerns about the amended form used by the PCT.

3) The PCT had to be reminded to make the amendments to the assessment form recommended by the Healthcare Commission.

[You complain that you had to ask the Healthcare Commission to follow this up four months later as you were unable to pursue your complaint to the Ombudsman until this had been resolved.]

4) The Healthcare Commission advised you that they could only look at how information was collected and provided by the PCT; not at how this affected your son personally. You have since been advised by a solicitor that this is incorrect. You told me that you wrote to Mr Palmer at the Healthcare Commission to clarify this, but have not received a satisfactory response.

5) The Healthcare Commission has closed your complaint, but the amended assessment form is

ANDREW'S STORY

an interim measure which the PCT has failed to finalise.

6) The PCT and the Healthcare Commission have both failed to answer your question about why your son is not deemed to be medically vulnerable when he has five major health problems, including conditions covered by the DDA.

You told me that the outcome you hope for is an acknowledgement and apology from the PCT that they gave inaccurate information about medical vulnerability.

I have studied the Healthcare Commission's file and your correspondence and note that since we received their papers you have been in more recent correspondence with the Healthcare Commission. I have written to the Healthcare Commission to ask for copies of more recent correspondence and requested that they keep me informed of any further communication relevant to your complaint. I have also written to the PCT to advise them of your complaint to the Ombudsman and to request an update on the current procedures for assessing medical vulnerability in relation to housing applications. Once I have received and studied these responses I will advise you of the next stage of my investigation.

Brenda Prentice

I now turn to the other questions and issues which you have raised. I have discussed these with my manager and can advise you that:

a) Your complaint with the Parliamentary Ombudsman cannot be investigated jointly because the complaints are at different stages: your Parliamentary complaint has been investigated and a report has been issued, whereas your Health Service complaint is in the early stages of investigation. We may consult the Parliamentary file for any information we need, but we cannot conduct a joint investigation.

b) Your complaint/question about what information the Healthcare Commission requested from the Office of the Deputy Prime Minister cannot form part of this investigation. This is because the Ombudsman can only investigate matters which have been through the complaints process. You will need to address this concern directly with the Healthcare Commission.

c) You asked what redress would be appropriate if your complaints about the PCT were upheld and whether any form of compensation could be considered because you have spent over £8,000 converting part of your home to provide appropriate accommodation for your son. I have noted this in your case file, but am unable to comment on questions of compensation at this stage of the investigation.

The other questions you have raised deal specifically with the Healthcare Commission's management of your case which do not form part of this investigation. I think you may have confused the Healthcare Commission and the Ombudsman's Office (I note that you initially sent correspondence to me at the Healthcare Commission's address by mistake). I can only suggest that any further queries relating to the Healthcare Commission are put directly to them. Your complaints about the Healthcare Commission which are being investigated by the Ombudsman's Office are as detailed in points 3 to 6 above.

I hope this letter has clarified things for you. I will keep you informed of progress with my investigation. In the meantime, if you have any further queries please feel free to telephone Dr Hayes on the number given above or to email me directly.

Yours sincerely,

Sarah Hopkins

Associate Investigator

Brenda Prentice

19 January 2007

From Parliamentary and Health Service Ombudsman.

Dear Andrew,

Your complaints against the former Taunton Deane Primary Trust and the Healthcare Commission

1. I am writing to let you know my draft findings and conclusions on your complaint against the former Taunton Deane Primary Care Trust (the PCT) 1 and the Healthcare Commission (the Commission). My draft report is based upon the documentation and advice available to me at this time; you, the PCT and the Commission now have an opportunity to provide comments on this draft before the report is finalised. I have not included in this report a reference to every detail examined in the course of the investigation, but I am satisfied that nothing significant has been overlooked.

Complaint against the PCT

2. When you spoke to my colleague Ms Hopkins on 19 May 2006, you explained that your son, had suffered from Pancreatitis since his teens and had his pancreas removed in his early twenties. He

suffers from brittle diabetes and chronic pain. He was unable to work and applied to Taunton Deane Borough Council (the Council) for housing assistance. In July 2003 an assessment was made of whether he had priority for housing due to medical vulnerability. As part of that assessment the Council sought information from the PCT, and the PCT sought information from your son's GP. The Council subsequently decided that your son did not fit the criteria for medical vulnerability and he was refused priority for social housing. You and your son were devastated by this, and you have complained about the PCT's role in the assessment.

3. You have explained that your main concern was the form used by the PCT to assess medical vulnerability in relation to the application for social housing; the PCT had been aware that the form was inadequate a year before your son's assessment. You complained also that the PCT's assessment was based simply on a GP's completion of two tick boxes on this form and the PCT did not review the medical records or seek expert opinion from the specialist who was treating him.

4. You explained that the outcome which you were seeking from this investigation was an acknowledgement and an apology that the PCT

had given inaccurate information to the housing department about his medical vulnerability.

Documentary Evidence

5. On 8 July 2003 the PCT received a request from the Council asking whether this man could be considered vulnerable under the terms of the 1996 Housing Act and on 9 July the PCT sent a standard request to the GP to assess medical vulnerability in relation to housing. The GP ticked both boxes to indicate that he did not suffer from any medical condition which interfered with mobility and did not suffer from any mental health problems which would put him in the category of vulnerability.

6. Having been contacted by you, the Council's Homelessness and Advice Officer wrote to the PCT asking for a medical opinion on your concerns that your son had serious medical problems and was receiving high rate disability living allowance which did indicate medical vulnerability. The PCT again sought the opinion of the Dr. Harrison.

7. The GP wrote to the PCT confirming that Andrew suffered from severe chronic Pancreatitis, was taking quantities of opiates for analgesia and was unable to work. However, the GP advised that according to the guidelines for assessing

medical vulnerability in relation to housing application he did not consider that Andrew satisfied either of the relevant criteria; mobility or mental health problems. That information was sent to the Council's housing department.

8. The PCT's Complaints Manager's letter to you of 5 August 2004 included:

'I am advised that a completed form was received from Taunton Deane Borough Council in respect of Andrew and this, together with a covering letter as described above, was forwarded to the GP on 9 July 2003. The form was returned directly to Taunton Deane Borough Council. It should be understood that [the PCT] has no input into the information supplied by the GP. It should also be emphasised that decisions regarding allocation of housing are solely within the responsibility of the Borough Council and not the PCT'.

9. In a letter to this Office, dated 13 June 2006, the PCT's Acting Chief Executive said that the process at the time of the complaint regarding the PCT's response to requests for assessment of medical vulnerability had been set out in their letter to you of 5 August 2004 (see paragraph 8 above). He explained that, because the PCT did not have direct clinical contact with Andrew on a routine basis, the assessment was passed to his GP for completion. He continued:

'The PCT's Director of Public Health would have reviewed the information provided by the general practitioner in the event that there was any conflict or confusion in the response but there would have been no evident reason to have queried the response in this case …

'… the form and associated process used at the time … was based on a form and process that had been used between Taunton Deane Borough Council and the former Somerset Health Authority's Health Protection Unit prior to the inception of the [PCT].

'The PCT followed the existing procedure in its provision of advice at that time and does not accept that this process was "inadequate" or that it had been identified as such a year before this incident. Clearly, there is always scope to improve the way in which such things are done and there have been changes to the form and subsequently the process since this time but I am satisfied from the investigation carried out by the Trust that the procedure was followed appropriately at the time.

ANDREW'S STORY

'... the PCT requested an assessment of Andrew's condition from his general practitioner, who would be best placed to advise on his medical vulnerability. At the time of the incident, the Trust had no reason to query the assessment provided and responded to the local authority accordingly. ...

'The PCT has acknowledged to that there were some shortcomings in its handling of the complaint and I reiterate the Trust's apology for these failings. However, I am satisfied that the Trust followed correctly the existing process at the time of the original application and that there has been an active review of the system which is used to consider these issues.'

Findings

10. You have complained that the PCT provided the Council with inadequate information on which to assess your son's eligibility for priority housing. The responsibility for obtaining adequate information about an applicant's medical vulnerability in relation to an application for housing rests with the Council. It follows that the Council is also responsible for asking the correct questions to enable it to obtain sufficient information on which to reach an informed

decision. It was also for the Council to determine the criteria for assessing eligibility for priority housing. The PCT was not responsible for assessing your son; its role in this matter was simply to obtain information to pass on to the Council to enable it to determine whether he fitted those criteria. The PCT did not hold that information itself and it forwarded the request for information to the GP. The PCT has said that it followed the procedure in place at the time; and explained that that procedure had been used between the Council and the former Somerset Health Authority's Health Protection Unit prior to the inception of the PCT, and was accepted as adequate by the Council. I am satisfied that the PCT correctly followed agreed procedures to provide information to the Council's housing department; it was for the Council to set the criteria for priority housing, and to assess eligibility. I do not uphold the complaint.

11. You are concerned that the assessment form that the PCT sent to the GP was inadequate. The PCT has explained that the form used in July 2003 had been inherited from the Health Protection Unit of the former Somerset Health Authority, and was accepted by the Council at that time. I do not see how the PCT can be held responsible for a form which its predecessors had designed and which had been deemed acceptable by the Council at the time of its inception and since. That said I

note that when the Commission considered your complaint it felt that the form was too restrictive and requested that the PCT revise the form, in conjunction with the Council if necessary.

12. You have complained that the PCT had to be reminded to make the amendments to the assessment form. The Commission's letter to the PCT was dated 22 March 2005 and the PCT's Chief Executive wrote to the Commission on 11 April 2005 to confirm that the PCT's Director for Public Health was in contact with the Council to review the process and form used to obtain a medical opinion in relation to an assessment of medical vulnerability.

13. On 9 August 2005 the Commission wrote to the PCT expressing concern that neither it nor your had received further information and concern that assessments were still being undertaken using the old form. The PCT responded on 15 August, confirming that the amendments had been made and put in place while the PCT and the Council revised their local assessment procedures. The PCT apologised for the delay in amending the form, confirming that this had been due to discussions between the PCT and the Council. The response was copied to you. On 20 October 2005 the Commission wrote to advise you that the PCT had complied with its recommendation and the case was closed.

14. In response to the Ombudsman, the PCT's Acting Chief Executive wrote:

> *'I acknowledge that there was a regrettable delay in the process leading to the amendment of the form, as recommended by the Commission. The PCT has acknowledged and apologised for this delay, although, again, it is important to be clear that the form had to be agreed between the parties involved and other parties were not bound by the Commission's deadlines.'*

> *'The amended form has now been almost entirely superseded by the new system used by the local authority for obtaining opinion on medical vulnerability. Taunton Deane Borough Council now uses a private company … as the source for its assessment of applicants' medical vulnerability.'*

15. The PCT has explained the reason for the delay in amending the assessment form and has apologised for this. I am satisfied that there is no outstanding injustice in relation to this matter. You have said that the Commission recommended that the PCT amend the form in consultation with Shelter and failed to do so. However, the

ANDREW'S STORY

Commission's letter of 22 March 2005, in which it set out its recommendation, does not mention Shelter; it says that the PCT should revise the form in conjunction with the Council, if necessary. I understand that Shelter was involved in discussions on the form and made comments, but there was no requirement that they be involved, nor was the PCT obliged to accept any comments that Shelter may have made.

Complaint against the Commission

16. You complained that the Commission had advised you incorrectly that it could look only at how information was collected and provided by the PCT; not at how this affected Andrew personally.

17. Following receipt of copy of the PCT's response to the Commission's recommendations (dated 15 August 2005), you e-mailed one of the Commission's case managers (the first Case Manager) to ask for clarification of number of points. The first Case Manager responded in an e-mail dated 18 August, in which she stated:

> 'For the purposes of progressing your complaint, I can only look at the changes to the form. If you are dissatisfied with the changes they have made you need to formally request the Healthcare Commission to look again at this aspect of

your complaint. This should be done with 2 months of the date of [the PCT's Chief Executive's] *letter.'*

18. Following a second complaint to the Commission, on 27 January 2006 you sent an email to the new case manager (the second Case Manager) to advise him that you had spoken to a solicitor who had said that the Commission could look at how a person has been affected by events. You complained that the first Case Manager had told you that she could only look at how information was collected, not how it had affected your son.

19. The second Case Manager replied on the same date advising that he would need further information before he could comment, but that if you felt that the Commission should have considered other issues, you had the right to ask them formally to reconsider.

20. The Commission's response to the Ombudsman stated that it can consider how issues affect an individual, and that the first and second Case Managers had tried to explain this to you, adding: *'Unfortunately it is evident that there still remains confusion and we apologise for this.'*

Finding

ANDREW'S STORY

21. There is no evidence that the Commission told you that it could not look at how your son was affected by the issues about which you had complained. It was only in response to further questions from you **after** the case had been closed by the Commission that the first Case Manager advised you that, for the purpose of progressing the complaint, she could only look at changes to the form. This was because that was the only area of complaint about which the Commission had made a recommendation.

22. I believe that you may have misunderstood what the original Case Manager told you. The second Case Manager could not clarify this because he was not aware of the context in which the comments had been made. In its response to this Office, the Commission has apologised for the confusion and have explained the context of their recommendation about the process by which GPs are asked to assess medical vulnerability.

23. It is evident that your confusion about whether the Commission could look into how your son was affected by the issues you complained about was not clarified by its Case Managers, although they did make attempts to do so. I uphold the complaint against the Commission to this limited extent, but I note that the Commission have now explained their position and apologised to you so I shall leave the matter there.

24. Finally, you have complained that the PCT and the Commission have failed to answer your question as to why Andrew was not deemed to be medically vulnerable when he has five major health problems, including conditions covered by the Disability Discrimination Act. However, neither the PCT nor the Commission can determine whether a person is medically vulnerable in relation to housing legislation. Therefore I do not criticise them for not answering your question to them about his medical vulnerability; indeed they would have been acting beyond their role had they attempted to do so. I should add that the Ombudsman, too, cannot answer your question.

Conclusion

25. I hope that you will be reassured that your concerns about the actions of the PCT and the Commission have now been thoroughly and independently reviewed, and that no major shortcomings have been identified. The PCT is no longer involved in the process of assessing medical vulnerability and that seems to me to be a good thing. They were, in effect, acting only as messengers, and direct contact between those doing the assessment (the Council) and an

applicant's clinicians will prevent problems of this nature occurring again.

26. With regard to your fundamental underlying issue of concern – the lack of priority which the Council have given to your son's application for housing – that is not something in which the Health Service Ombudsman could become involved.

27. As I noted above, this is a draft report and you, the PCT and the Commission now have an opportunity to comment on it before it is finalised. Any comments you have should be put in writing to arrive here by 5 February. If I do not hear from you by then I will assume that you are content with the report. Once I have considered any comments I receive I hope to be in a position to finalise the report.

Yours sincerely,

David Herbert

Senior Investigation Officer
Health and Parliamentary Ombudsman

1 Taunton Deane Primary Care Trust was dissolved on 30 September 2006 and replaced by the new Somerset Primary Care Trust.

2 The actions of the GP are the subject of a separate investigation.

3 The actions of the Council are outside the Ombudsman's jurisdiction.

ANDREW'S STORY

**To Parliamentary and Health Service
Ombudsman**

24th January 2007

Millbank Tower
Millbank

Dear Mr. Herbert,

I have your letter of the 19th January. I take it that you are responding on behalf of Dr. Hayes and Ms. Hopkins? It feels like every time I hear from someone, it's a different name. Oh well, at least I keep you people in work!

Please bear in mind what my complaint was. 'The PCT should put their own house in order so that sick people do not have to go through the trauma of having to make a complaint'. (Or words to that meaning)

1. Please send me the file which you have based your draft conclusion on.

2. Andrew suffers from brittle diabetes and is insulin dependant, he suffers from chronic pain for which he takes prescribed morphine, he takes Senner to relieve the effects of morphine. He suffers from mal-absorption for which he takes Creon, projectile vomiting for which he takes

Motillium and depression for which he takes Amitriptyline. He has Nexium to reduce stomach acid and to make a better environment for Creon to work. He takes vitamin supplements A & D.

He was sacked from his job (illegally, case fought and won). He applied to the Council for assistance when he became homeless and the Council asked for information from the PCT. Dr M from the PCT approached Andrew's then GP who put two ticks on in a tick box form! Andrew could not complain about this doctor at the time as he still had to attend his practice. When he did complain to the Ombudsman he was told that he was out of time and too late to complain.

We were devastated that with all his medical problems, Andrew was said not to be medically vulnerable. What was Dr. Morkane thinking of by not questioning that opinion? As a doctor himself, alarm bells should have rung and he should have contacted Andrew's specialists as I had requested, but he didn't. Ultimately the result of this opinion is that Andrew can 'live on the streets without detriment the same as any other homeless person'. Dr. Morkane must have been aware of that, it is printed on the form, in any case it is secondary to commonsense! How could Andrew keep insulin in a fridge, needles clean and morphine in a safe place when living on the streets? As a doctor and Director of Public

ANDREW'S STORY

Health, Dr Morkane would know that without a permanent address that there could be no prescriptions and that without medication Andrew's condition is terminal. The housing issues are secondary to this miscarriage of justice and common sense. We have housed Andrew, so housing does not come into this now. It is the medical information we complained about, it was just incomprehensible!

3. Our main concern is that the doctor involved (Dr. Morkane) did not know what is medical vulnerability! Therefore he should not have given the PCT's opinion, where ever they got it from. Just as ignorance is not tolerated in law braking, ignorance is no excuse in this case. The judge said that the information should be reliable, it was not. How could it be when you consider how it was obtained! **With two tick boxes!** If Dr. Morkane had thought about it, instead of simply backing a fellow professional, he would have spoken to the specialists involved as I asked. Why didn't he? Was it arrogance, he thought he knew better then me?

4. When people make mistakes and we are all human and do make mistakes, an apology is what civilised people do! It would have made Andrew feel better about himself instead of driving him further down the road of no self confidence and furthering his depression.

5. The form sent by the PCT to Dr. Harrison clearly states the 'critical test' which is, 'whether the applicant is less able to fend for him/her self so that she/he will suffer injury or detriment, in circumstances where a less vulnerable person would be able to cope without harmful effects'. Any doctor should know that chronic pain does interfere with mobility (Andrew is often paralyzed with pain) and that depression is a well recognised mental condition. I will return to depression later. Again alarm bells should have rang for Dr. Morkane but they didn't, why?   What sort of a doctor is he? Was he qualified and fit to do the job of Public Health Director?

6. By now the PCT should have been asking questions about this doctor, but they didn't. They said there had been no complaints made about him, **which is not true**. The PCT did not consult the specialists involved with Andrew's care. The GP was wrong in ticking both boxes, probably because he never visited Andrew at home and simply didn't know how he was affected by his hidden disabilities. I doubt he had ever come across another case of Pancreatitis in his career and he wasn't known for 'effort' in the village. I could send you dozens of affidavits as to how this disease affects people, **do you want me to**? Will it make any difference?

ANDREW'S STORY

Disability Living Allowance is no measure of housing need, sometimes it is paid to people who are in work. The Council said Dr. Morkane had written to the DLA saying Andrew was not entitled to DLA. **Why was that done?** It was an un-necessary and unkind thing to do, but not as unkind and un-necessary as not withdrawing the letter. That has added to Andrew's distress! (1)

7. You know the critical test; I ask you, is the GP's opinion viable? The information was sent to the Council **VIA** the PCT. The PCT sent the information to the Council and they should have seen it was correct, ignorance is no excuse. The PCT cannot hide behind, 'it was sent direct to the council', it was not. Even if it was, they are responsible to see that their doctors perform properly.

8. The form was returned to Maggie Haworth at the PCT. The PCT are responsible for doctor's professional behaviour, what ever Ms. Pope was advised, **do we know who advised her?** The decision the council made on Andrew's housing was based on information supplied by the PCT, it should have been reliable, it was not. Ms. Pope states in her letter of 5 Aug 04, that '*allocation of housing is solely within the responsibility of Taunton Deane Borough Council and not the PCT.* And yet in a letter to Ms Wray on the 15th August 05 Mr. Colgan states*, 'I can confirm, however, that*

the PCT remains willing to review Andrew's priority points on the housing list should we be asked to do so by the housing department at T/D council'. (2)

Ms. Pope's letter to me of the 5th Aug 04 also states that, '*I can only apologise (*for ignoring letters*) and would wish to assure you that all relevant staff have been reminded of the need to reply promptly to correspondence'.* She continues, along with Jan Hull to ignore letters from me! It may be that I ask inconvenient questions as far as they are concerned, but she said letters would be answered in 2 working days! They are not. As advised by Dr. Hayes, I have made another complaint to the Commission!

9. A. 'no evident reason to have queried the response in this case' **WHY?** What university did Dr. Morkane qualify in if he could find nothing wrong with the doctor's findings? Why was he put through the PCT's 'Poor Performance' programme if there was nothing wrong? He has since taken early retirement due to some unidentified mystery illness). If the *'Director of Public Health would have reviewed the information provided'*, the form did go to the Trust then.

9.b. And the reason for changing from the former SHA to the PCT was....? Perhaps the PCT should have not simply taken over procedures without looking at them first!

9.c The PCT do not accept that this process was 'inadequate', so why had there been discussions with Shelter and a promise made to them that the form would be altered a year before? Not until Ms. Wray directed the PCT to make changes were they made and then not willingly or with any haste! **Do you want me to supply affidavits from Shelter?** Ms Hull is satisfied that the appropriate procedure was followed. I know where she is coming from....! The procedure was inadequate, not fit for purpose, as Ms. Wray found and Andrew has suffered from it,

9 d Dr. Morkane said in a letter to me that there are more important issues than medical vulnerability. In spite of asking many times, I was never told **what they were**. I thought the PCT were asked about the council's need to know about the 'nature and extent of the disability or illness which might render Andrew vulnerable'. Dr Morkane letter of the 13 Oct 03 say's otherwise. (3)

9e Yes, they did apologise for not answering letters in a timely fashion. That was not the main complaint. Jan Hull maybe satisfied that they '*followed correctly the existing process at the time...*' **I am not**. Did their existing procedure include telling the DLA that Andrew was not entitled to the DLA benefit? Did it exclude asking specialists for an opinion? Did it include writing to me to say 'there are more important things to consider than his medical condition'? Did it include not telling us what they were? If she is satisfied, then I have questions about her ability to do her job! Reviewing the system does not help us, a meaningful apology would.

10. As the judge said, where advice is sought it must be reliable and having taken advice it would be dereliction not to accept it. The Council explained to Dr. Morkane that they *needed to know the nature and extent of the illness or disability which might render Andrew vulnerable'*. How can that be done with two tick boxes? The Council could not be clearer in asking the question. The PCT cannot wriggle out of their responsibility by saying the council didn't ask the right question! That is absurd. This bat and ball between all authorities gives the ideal opportunity to pass the buck, well the buck must stop with someone! I think it is the job of the Ombudsman to find some justice for Andrew in these issues, unless of course there are more important things than he is, to be considered.

In a letter, no date, Ms. Wray said, *'I have decided to take no further action as I am satisfied that at the time of Andrew's application… the practice was not giving cause for concern'.* The PCT may have led her to that conclusion but it was not correct as Ms. Nelson demonstrated, but then she no longer works for the PCT! Their procedure for identifying problems had failed, there were many complaints, but the department for dealing with them didn't know. It was common knowledge in the village that all was not well with the practice; the numbers of people who left the list should have rung alarm bells, why did the PCT ask patients in the circular I have provided to you, for opinions on the practice! It was unfortunate for some patients that they could not move to a different list, depending on where they lived.

The PCT **was** responsible for the information it gave, **the judge said so!**

In his letter to me (Number 3) 13th Oct 03. Dr. Morkane say's in the second sentence, the **medical** opinion of Andrew has not changed. Actually the Disability Rights Act says that where someone is covered by that act, they are for housing purposes covered! But Dr. Morkane is giving an opinion; I thought he only passed information? He also say's that there are more important things to consider than Andrew's medical condition, but we don't know what, but Dr. Morkane considers them more important, who asked him for that opinion?

By December 2005 we find that Dr. Morkane does not have the *'practical experience of reviewing adequacy of an individual's accommodation'*. No passing of information here then. Do not forget that Andrew had no home at the time of the application he was being made homeless. Therefore Dr. Morkane's experience of reviewing accommodation is not the question.(4) The question is, can Andrew live on the streets without detriment…

My complaint was not about a form! That was Ms. Wray's complaint! What is the complaint that you do not uphold?

11. It was the PCT who were 'collecting evidence' and up to them to do it properly, not for the council to tell them how to do it, that is a red herring which the Commission saw through.

12. Yes, you see I was waiting to go to the Ombudsman with my complaint but I couldn't do that until the PCT had complied.

13. No, the PCT confirmed that interim amendments had been made as directed by the Commission; a final amendment was never made. Why did I have to chase this up? The ombudsman's lady, Mrs. Olrunniwo, I think it was, would not let me proceed until this had been completed. So Ms Wray said I could proceed to

the Ombudsman and Mrs Olrunniwo said I
couldn't!

14. Not me governor, them!
The amended form is *'almost entirely superseded'*
(!) What does this mean, do they now pick and
choose who gets sent to Nowmedical and who do
not? No one told me that the PCT had
recommended Nowmedical! I have asked for an
opinion from the Commission regarding the
recommendation by the PCT of this firm, is this
ethical? But as usual there is no answer, I spend
years getting, no answer!   I understand that
there are now questions being asked in
Parliament about this firm, will you carry on letting
PCT's recommend them?

15. If the form had been amended when the PCT
told Shelter it would be, then Andrew would not
have been disadvantaged by it. Ms. Wray said
she wanted interim amendments to the form **so
that no one else would be disadvantaged by it**.
You are easily satisfied that there is no injustice!
Why was Andrew's disadvantage not considered?

Shelter was involved the previous year and has
not heard from the PCT or Council since then. I
did ask who is supposed to have made contact
with Shelter as they wanted to know, but as usual,
no answer. Just a figment of some ones
imagination! Unless you can tell me who?

16. This is correct.

17. Confused, yes I am! If the Commission looked at the way information was collected and provided and **CAN** look at how it affects an individual, why wasn't it done? It was the way in which information was collected that adversely effected Andrew, but nothing was said about this other than, (first case manager) *we cannot look at how it has affected an individual*! I'm still confused, can it or can it not look at how it affected Andrew?

18. It was when I saw my solicitor about something completely different that he asked how Andrew was and I told him what had been said. He said that was wrong! Will you look at how Andrew was affected then?

19. Second case manager had all the information, what more did he want? He didn't know! I still don't know! Most unhelpful, but then I guess he didn't know himself! Do you know?

20 Thank them for the apology, what I really would like to know is why they can't answer me in language that I can understand? If they can consider how things affect an individual, why didn't they?

ANDREW'S STORY

21 Why do the Commission think I was complaining? If it was the case that they could look at this, why didn't they do it, or inform me they could? They informed me they couldn't and I believed them! Why do you think I discussed it with my solicitor saying they will not look at how it has affected Andrew? Why do they act in such a confusing way? I think you are telling me that they could look at how this affected Andrew but they didn't, or are you saying I didn't ask the right question or make the right complaint? Please ask them to look at it now. When do you think the case was closed?

22. I don't think I am stupid, why am I so confused? Could it be the way this whole case has been handled? If I misunderstood the original case manager why was that? What did she think I was complaining about? As an ordinary member of the public I have found this whole procedure a nightmare, made worse by the complexities of the case which I'm not convinced you all understand. It seems that a bit of it is latched on to and the others bits are ignored as they don't fit in. I can't believe you are now telling me they can look at how Andrew was disadvantaged, why didn't they?

23. Demonstrate how they tried to clarify this with me! Can you tell me where I can find this apology and who it was from. Each time I receive a communication it's from another person! Can you

be surprised at my confusion? Why are you leaving the matter there? If they can look at how Andrew was disadvantaged then they should do so. If they can't, please explain why?

24. I did not ask 'in relation to housing legislation! I asked "If five major health conditions don't make you medically vulnerable, what does?" And I would like an answer! I'm not asking you about housing regulations, I'm asking you about medical matters, isn't that what you are there for?

25. You hope I am reassured! No I am not. The review seems to me to take advantage of the complexities of this case and to give the opportunity for passing the buck! Where is justice for Andrew in all this? It seems to have got lost on the way. All the Director of Public Health had to do was use his brain and think to himself as a doctor, is what Dr. Harrison telling me correct, how can a brittle diabetic live on the streets, but he was too keen to join the merry throng in destroying Andrew. He just joined the band wagon. Andrew's new GP, or in fact the GP he had as a child, wrote to Dr. Morkane in support of Andrew after Andrew came home to live with us. We thought he would be home temporarily but his independence was taken from him and he must live with us permanently now. The GP's letter was ignored as was Andrew's gastro specialist opinion. It would have been inconvenient to listen to them,

someone might have had to get off their bums and help Andrew, we can't have that!

26. My fundamental underlying concern is the inability of the PCT to do a proper job in relation to supplying information. Having realised that they were wrong, the PCT are simply facing it out, not trying to put matters right. This is not about a housing issue, it is about how the PCT works and how it deals with their mistakes and the most vulnerable members of society. I came to you for justice and Dr. Hayes asked me to trust her!

My Conclusion.

With all that has gone on I have looked further into this whole affair. After Andrew had been ill for five years there was a new doctor at the hospital. He informed a hospital in Plymouth where Andrew had gone as a student that Andrew was an alcoholic and drug addict. **I would have noticed if Andrew had been an alcoholic at 15!** Or his house master would have!

I found this letter in a bundle sent by the previous GP to a hospital in Liverpool. We had gone there for a second opinion at their request. We had a particularly hostile reception and we wondered why we had wasted our money going to see this doctor, what was it all about. The Liverpool doctor is researching on behalf of EuroPac and sees anyone he can from all over the country. I asked to see the referral note and my request was ignored until I sent a solicitors letter! It did explain a lot, including why Andrew often seemed to have poor or sometimes hostile treatment in hospital. I have written to this doctor recently and he has apologised. It does not undo all the harm it has caused, but we will not sue him, he was man enough to accept our criticism and apologised! The PCT could learn from him! Why the doctor had to send a letter dating from 1991, I don't know, there were many other letters pre dating that on the file which were fair and not damming.

Over the Christmas period Andrew has been falling and we have had to take him to the hospital or GP to be sewn up on six occasions. We now know that he is self harming, not falling, although he has no remembrance of it. The psychiatrist says he is in a psychological 'fugue' state. He is so enraged at what has happened to him and he has no way of venting is feelings, that he takes it out on himself, but puts it out of his mind. He has no memory of it. Suicide is a real possibility again. If he should succeed, I will make sure that the authorities know exactly what has happened to him over the years and why he did it. He has been let down by all those who should have been there to help him. I will call it, hounded to death by those who should have helped.

ANDREW'S STORY

If you don't believe me you can ask Dr. Ahmed at Cheddon Rd.

I came to the authorities for justice, but there hasn't been any. Guidelines also ask authorities to follow the spirit of the law, not just the law and you can do that. There has only been a certain arrogant attitude, not uncommonly used towards undesirable people. I have seen it before, used on homeless people at the homeless hostel.

You can make a difference. I would like answers to my questions, I think that is the least you can do for us.

Yours sincerely,

Brenda Prentice

From
Parliamentary and Health Service Ombudsman

8th February 2007

Dear Andrew,

Your complaint against the former Taunton Deane Primary Care Trust and the Health Care Commission

1. Thank you for your letter about the draft report of the investigation into your complaints against the former Taunton Deane Health Care Trust (PCT) and the Healthcare Commission (the Commission). Acting with the authorisation of the Ombudsman in accordance with paragraph 12 of Schedule 1 to the Health Service Commission Act 1993, this letter is my report to you of the results of the investigation and my finds. I have not included in the report a reference to every detail examined in the course of the investigation, but I am satisfied that nothing significant has been overlooked.

2. As I explained on the phone on the 25th January, I have worked on your complaint in collaboration with Ms. Hopkins, who is one of the Ombudsman's Associate Investigators, and Dr. Hayes, Investigating Manager. Dr. Hayes has seen and approved this report.

ANDREW'S STORY

3. I note your point that the essence of your complaint was that the PCT should 'put it's own house in order', As you are aware, this investigation has not identified any significant short comings in the actions of the PCT. Moreover, the PCT no longer exists as a distinct entity and the process of assessing priority housing need in your area no longer involves even the new PCT. That being the case, I can see no merit in making any criticisms of, or recommendations to, the PCT.

4. You asked to have access to the Ombudsman's file about your complaint: I shall pass that request to the Ombudsman's Data Protection/ Freedom of Information team, who will contact you shortly.

5. You make a number of points in your letter questioning the actions and competence of Dr. Morkane and Dr. Harrison, the status of Andrew's claim for disability living allowance; and the involvement of Nowmedical and Shelter. As I am sure you will appreciate, this investigation concerned only the actions of the PCT in dealing with the council's request for information about Andrew, and the investigation of that by the Commission. It is not the role of the Ombudsman to consider more general issues such as those which you have raised.

6. You asked about the apology from the Commission – that was conveyed to me by the Commissions Senior Complaints Policy and Reconsideration manager; I have quoted from his letter in paragraph 26 below.

7. You concluded your letter by describing the difficulties which you and your family are facing because of your son's problems. I was sorry to learn of your predicament and I hope that he is now getting appropriate medical care.

Complaint against the PCT

8. When you spoke to my colleague Ms. Hopkins on 19th May 2006, you explained that your son, had suffered from Pancreatitis since his teens and has had his pancreas removed in his early twenties. He suffers from brittle diabetes and chronic pain. He was unable to work and applied to Taunton Deane Borough Council (the council) for housing assistance. In July 2003 an assessment was made of whether he had priority for housing due to medical vulnerability. As part of that assessment the council sought information from the PCT, and the PCT sought information from your son's then GP. The Council subsequently decided that your son did not fit the criteria for medical vulnerability and he was refused priority for social housing. You and you son were devastated by this, and you have

complained about the PCT's role in the assessment.

9. You have explained that your main concern was the form used by the PCT to assess medical vulnerability in relation to the application for social housing; the PCT had been aware that the form was inadequate a year before your son's assessment. You complained also that the PCT's assessment was based simply on the GP's completion of two tick boxes on this form and the PCT did not review the medical records or seek expert opinion from the specialist who was treating your son.

10. You explained that the outcome which you were seeking from this investigation was an acknowledgement and an apology that the PCT had given inaccurate information to the housing department about Andrew's medical vulnerability.

Documentary Evidence

11. On 8 July 2003 the PCT received a request from the council asking whether Andrew could be considered vulnerable under the terms of the 1996 Housing Act and on the 9th July the PCT sent a standard request to the GP to assess Andrew's medical vulnerability in relation to housing. The GP ticked both boxes to indicate information to the

housing department about Andrew's medical vulnerability.

12. Having been contacted by you, the council's homelessness and advice officer wrote to the PCT asking for a medical opinion on your concerns that Andrew had serious medical problems and was receiving high rate disability living allowance which did indicate medical vulnerability. The PCT again sought the opinion of the GP.

13. Dr. Harrison wrote to the PCT confirming that Andrew suffered from severe chronic Pancreatitis, was taking quantities of opiates for analgesia and was unable to work. However, the GP advised that according to the guidelines for assessing medical vulnerability in relation to housing application he did not consider that Andrew satisfied either of the relevant criteria: mobility or mental health problems. That information was sent to the council's housing department.

14. The PCT's complaints manager's letter to you of the 5th August 2004 included:

'I am advised that a completed form was received from Taunton Deane Borough Council in respect of Andrew and this, together with a covering letter as described above, was forwarded to Andrew's GP on the 9th July 2003. The ... form was returned directly to Taunton Deane Borough Council. It

should be understood that the PCT has no input into the information supplied by the GP. It should also be emphasised that decisions regarding allocation of housing are solely within the responsibility of Taunton Deane Borough Council and not the PCT'.

15. In a letter to this Office, dated 13th June, the PCT's Acting Chief Executive said that the process at the time of the complaint regarding the PCT's response to requests for assessment of medical vulnerability had been set out in their letter to you of 5th August 2004 (see paragraph 8 above). He explained that, because the PCT did not have direct clinical contact with Andrew on a routine basis, the assessment was passed to his GP for completion. He continued:

'The PCT's Director of Public Health would have reviewed the information provided by the general practitioner in the event that there was any conflict or confusion in the response in this case…

…the form and associated process used at the time… was based on a form and process that had been used between Taunton Deane Borough Council and the former Somerset Health Authority's Health Protection unit prior to the inception of the PCT.

The PCT followed the existing procedure in it's provision of advice at that time and does not accept that this process was "inadequate" or that it had been identified as such a year before this incident. Clearly, there is always scope to improve the way in which such things are done and there have been changes to the form and subsequently the process since that time but I am satisfied from the investigation carried out by the Trust that the procedure was followed appropriately at the time.

...the PCT requested an assessment of Andrew's condition from his general practitioner, who would be best placed to advise on his medical vulnerability. At the time of the incident, the Trust had no reason to query the assessment provided and responded to the local authority accordingly...

...the PCT has acknowledged to you that there were some shortcomings in its handling of the complaint and I reiterate the Trusts apology for there failings. However, I am satisfied that the Trust followed correctly the existing process at the time of the original application and that there has been an active review of the system which is used to consider these issues.'

ANDREW'S STORY

Findings

16. You have complained that the PCT provided the council with inadequate information on which to assess your son's eligibility for priority housing. The responsibility for obtaining adequate information about an applicant's medical vulnerability in relation to an application for housing rests with the council. It follows that the council is also responsible for asking the correct questions to enable it to obtain sufficient information on which to reach an informed decision. It was also for the council to determine the criteria for assessing eligibility for priority housing. The PCT was not responsible for assessing your son; its role in this matter was simply to obtain information to pass on to the council to enable it to determine whether he fitted those criteria. The PCT did not hold that information itself and it forwarded the request for information to the GP. The PCT has said that it followed the procedure in place at the time; and explained that the procedure had been used between the council and the former Somerset Health Authority's Health Protection Unit prior to the inception of the PCT, and was accepted as adequate by the council. I am satisfied that the PCT correctly followed agreed procedures to provide information to the council's housing department; it was for the council to set the criteria

for priority housing, and to assess eligibility. I do not uphold the complaint.

17. You are concerned that the assessment form that the PCT sent to the GP was inadequate. The PCT has explained that the form used in July 2003 had been inherited from the Health Protection Unit of the former Somerset Health Authority, and was accepted by the council at that time. I do not see how the PCT can be held responsible for a form which its predecessors had designed and which had been deemed acceptable by the council at the time of its inception and since. That said, I note that when the Commission considered your complaint it felt that the form was too restrictive and requested that the PCT revise the form, in conjunction with the council if necessary.

18. You have complained that the PCT had to be reminded to make the amendments to the assessment from. The Commission's letter to the PCT was dated 22nd. March 2005 and the PCT Chief Executive wrote to the Commission on 11th April 2005 to confirm that the PCT's Director for Public Health was in contact with the council to review the process and form used to obtain a medical opinion in relation to an assessment of medical vulnerability.

19. On 9TH August 2005 the Commission wrote to the PCT expressing concern that neither it nor you

had received further information and concern that assessments were still being undertaken using the old form. The PCT responded on the 15th August, confirming that the amendments had been made and put in place while the PCT and the council revised their local assessment procedures. The PCT apologised for the delay in amending the form, confirming that this had been due to discussions between the PCT and the council. The response was copied to you. On the 20th October 2005 the Commission wrote to advise you that the PCT had complied with its recommendation and the case was closed.

20. In response to the Ombudsman, the PCT's Acting Chief Executive wrote:

'I acknowledge that there was a regrettable delay in the process leading to the amendment of the form, as recommended by the Commission. The PCT has acknowledged and apologised for this delay, although, again, it is important to be clear that the form had to be agreed between the parities involved and other parties were not bound by the Commission's deadlines.'

'The amended form has now been almost entirely superseded by the new system used by the local authority for obtaining opinion on medical vulnerability'. Taunton Deane Borough Council now uses a private company... as the source for

*its assessments of applicants' medical
vulnerability.'*

21. The PCT has explained the reason for the
delay in amending the assessment form and has
apologised for this. I am satisfied that there is no
outstanding injustice in relation to this matter. You
have said that the Commission recommended that
the PCT amend the form in consultation with
Shelter and failed to do so. However, the
Commission's letter of 22 March 2005, in which it
set out its recommendation, does not mention
Shelter; it says that the PCT should revise the
form in conjunction with the council, if necessary.
I understand that Shelter was involved in
discussions on the form and made comments, but
there was no requirement that they be involved,
nor was the PCT obliged to accept any comments
that Shelter may have made.

Complaint against the Commission

22. You complained that the Commission had
advised you incorrectly that it could look only at
how information was collected and provided by the
PCT; not at how this affected Andrew personally.

23. Following receipt of a copy of the PCT's
response to the Commission's recommendations
(dated August 2005), you emailed one of the
Commission's case managers (the first case

Manager) to ask for clarification of a number of points. The first Case manager responded in an email dated 18th August, in which she stated:

'For the purpose of progressing your complaint, I can only look at the changes to the form. If you are dissatisfied with the changes they have made you need to formally request the Healthcare Commission to look again at this aspect of your complaint. This should be done within 2 months of the date of the PCT's Chief Executive's letter.'

24. Following a second complaint to the Commission, on the 27th January 2006 you sent an email to the new case manager (the second case manager) to advise him that you had spoken to a solicitor who had said that the Commission could look at how a person has been affected by events. You complained that the first Case manager had told you that she could only look at how information was collected, not how it had affected your son.

25. The second Case Manager replied on the same day advising that he would need further information before he could comment, but that if you felt that the Commission should have considered other issues, you had the right to ask them formally to reconsider.

26. The Commission's response to the Ombudsman stated that it can consider how issues affect an individual, and that the first and second Case Managers had tried to explain this to you, adding: *'unfortunately it is evident that there still remains confusion and we apologise for this.'*

Findings

27. There is no evidence that the Commission told you that it could not look at how your son was affected by the issues about which you had complained. It was only in response to further questions from you **after** the case had been closed by the Commission that the first case Manager advised you that, for the purposes of progressing the complaint, she could only look at changes to the form. This was because that was the only area of complaint about which the Commission had made a recommendation.

28. I believe that you may have misunderstood what the original Case manager told you. The second Case Manager could not clarify this because he was not aware of the context in which the comments had been made. In its response to this office, the Commission has apologised for the confusion and have explained that context of their recommendation about the process by which GP's are asked to assess medical vulnerability.

29. It is evident that your confusion about whether that Commission could look into how your son was affected by the issues you complained about was not clarified by its Case Manager, although they did make an attempts to do so. I uphold the complaint against the Commission to this limited extent, but I note that the Commission have now explained their position and apologised to you so I shall leave it at the matter there.

30. Finally, you have complained that the PCT and the Commission have failed to answer your question as to why Andrew was not deemed to be medically vulnerable when he has five major health problems, including conditions covered by the Disability Discrimination Act. However, neither the PCT nor the Commission can determine whether a person is medically vulnerable in relation to housing legislation. Therefore I do not criticise them for not answering your question to them about Andrew's medical vulnerability; indeed they would be acting beyond their role had they attempted to do so. I should add that the Ombudsman, too, cannot answer your question.

Conclusion

31. I hope that you will be reassured that your concerns about the actions of the PCT and the Commission have now been thoroughly and independently reviewed, and that no major

shortcomings have been identified. The PCT is no longer involved in the process of assessing medical vulnerability and that seems to me to be a good thing. They were, in effect acting only acting as messengers, and direct contact between those doing the assessment (the council) and an applicant's clinicians will prevent problems of this nature occurring again.

32. With regard to your fundamental underlying issue of concern - the lack of priority which the council have given to your son's application for housing - that is not something in which the Health Service Ombudsman could become involved.

33. In accordance with statute I have sent a copy of this report to the Chief Executive of Somerset PCT, to the Healthcare Commission and to the secretary of State for Health.

Yours sincerely,

David Herbert   Senior
Investigating Officer.

ANDREW'S STORY

Letter to Ms. Shirlow 14th July 2003

Lettings and Advice Officer
Taunton Deane Borough Council
Taunton

Dear Ms. Shirlow,

In view for the information provided by this man's general practitioner, he would not appear to be medically vulnerable under the terms of the 1996 Housing Act.

Yours sincerely

Maggie Haworth

On behalf of Dr. Elaine Farmery, Consultant in Health Protection.
Taunton Deane Primary Care Trust

And on the same date. July 2003

To Ms. T Shirlow

Taunton Deane Borough Council
Taunton

Brenda Prentice

Dear Ms. Shirlow,

I refer to your query about this man's medical factors being considered in prioritisation for housing. I have now had a response from his GP and I consider that his present accommodation is adequate.

Yours sincerely,

Maggie Haworth

On behalf of Dr. Elaine Farmery, Consultant in Health Protection.
Taunton Deane Primary Care Trust.

ANDREW'S STORY

To Taunton Deane Borough Council. 20th December 2005

Dear Mrs. Mortimer

Further to your letter of 15th December and our telephone conversation this morning, I think it is best that you now use 'Nowmedical' to assess whether or not Andrew's current accommodation is unsuitable

As I explained to you I do not have practical experience of reviewing adequacy of an individual's accommodation in relation to their health needs. I think it is more appropriate you use health care professionals, such as Nowmedical who do this routinely.

I also mentioned to you that I will be leaving the Primary Care Trust on the 5th January 2006. If you address your further correspondence to the Director of Public Health' then appropriate action will be taken.

Yours sincerely,

Dr. Morkane
Director of Public Health

Brenda Prentice

The Local Government Ombudsman said that the second housing application should have had a separate medical assessment. It was belatedly performed by Nowmedical.

Dear Mr. Thornberry,

I refer to your letter 19th June 06 with the Now Medical report, which as you say, tests the reasonableness of the conclusion of Andrew's applications in April 04. As you say the report say's, no more points.

I trust there would be no objection to applying the same test of reasonableness to Andrew's other homeless application. We would pay the fee for Now Medical to look again at the issues involved, taking into consideration that the PCT have said they don't have the expertise to assess these issues.

You will remember that the judge did not uphold the medical decision, only the right of the Council to rely on it. As you know we cannot appeal the case having been denied leave to appeal. However it would help Andrew and me come to terms with this, if the test were upheld.

I understand from Ms. James that you are dealing with our complaint regarding the direction to the

ANDREW'S STORY

DLA from your Council, please tell me how long it
will take to deal with this and to answer the other
part of this letter.

Yours sincerely,

These issues have never been addressed!

Brenda Prentice

To the Chief Executive, Taunton Deane Borough Council

Dear Ms. James,

I made a complaint via the Deane web site. Eventually Mr. Thornberry made his usual answer to any communication I have with your Council. i.e., that has been covered by the Ombudsman and we have no further comment until their investigation is finished or something like that. I assured him that, having checked with the Ombudsman, their investigation is complete, but I have not heard from him since.

I would like you to ask your Ms. Shirlow to withdraw her request to the DLA that in her opinion Andrew is not entitled to DLA. She asked that her letter be left on file for the next review. As the doctor who gave such a false opinion has been taken through the PCT's 'poor performance' procedure (this was not connected with our complaint) and the Director of Public Health has left the PCT, I think it would be appropriate.

Please let me know as soon as possible, what your decision is.

Yours sincerely,

ANDREW'S STORY

And again!

Dear Ms. James,

The DLA are now looking at Andrew's renewal application of DLA.

I did ask that you let me know ASAP if you were going to ask
Ms. Shirlow to withdraw her remarks to the DLA. It is now 21 working days since my request, made on the 5th June. It is now the 5th July.

I have been told by Ms. Forester that Mr. Thornberry will arrange for a response at the earliest practical opportunity. Have you any idea what that means? Your web site says that I will receive a written response in 10 working days.

I was hoping that you, as the Chief Executive would take the lead in this issue and try to get it sorted out once and for all. I did phone to speak to you, but even your PA would not take my call, I was put through to
Mr. Thornberry's PA, even though I specifically asked that should not happen! What exactly is Mr. Thornberry's position in all this? Have you asked him to expedite this? A month does seem to me to be more than long enough to deal with this.

Please let me know by return if Ms. Shirlow will withdraw or not.

Yours sincerely,

This request was never answered and never dealt with!

There are 21 similar requests on several subjects not covered by the Ombudsman to Mr. Thornberry. None have been dealt with!

ANDREW'S STORY

From the Health Care Commission 3rd April 2007.

Dear Andrew,

I have now had the opportunity to review the file to your second complaint.

It appears the PCT was contacted following your claim 'that the PCT did not provide you with a copy of the finalised assessment form'. Having spoken to the PCT we have been advised that the form has now been superseded by a new procedure and that this had already been explained to you. The PCT were asked for a copy of the letter they sent to you explaining this.

In the meantime this point was covered in the recent Ombudsman's report and Mr. Luckie was therefore satisfied that you had been provided with an explanation.

I note that you feel that there are still outstanding issues that you wish the Healthcare Commission to review. I have read through the correspondence on file and believe that between his letters of January 4th and March 23rd. He has responded to all the issues you have raised. It would appear therefore that there is nothing for us to review.

Brenda Prentice

Yours sincerely

Ms. Wray
Senior Case Manager.

ANDREW'S STORY

May 29th 2007

From Healthcare Commission (second complaint)

Dear Andrew,

Re Reconsideration of the handling of your independent review.

Further to our telephone conversation of the 8th May 2007. I have now completed my reconsideration of the handling of the independent review by Mr. Luckie of your complaint about Taunton Deane Primary Care Trust.

In carrying out my reconsideration I have considered all the documentation gathered as part of the independent review. The reconsideration has focussed on the issues raised in your letter of complaint dated October 28th 2006 and in your letter of outstanding concerns dated January 8th 2007: your email of April 16th 2007 to Ms Wray and your emails of May 3rd 4th and 7th to myself. Where necessary I have referred to your previous independent review considered under other reviews. I have identified a degree of overlap with these issues. My decision has been approved by a senior colleague in accordance with the Healthcare Commission's quality assurance process.

Brenda Prentice

In your letter of January 8th 2007 you raised a number of concerns about the outcome of the independent review as set out in Mr. Luckie's decision letter of January 4th 2007. For ease of reference, I will refer to the issue numbers that you have used in your letter of January 8th 2007 to identify your specific concerns about the content of Mr. Luckie's letter.

ANDREW'S STORY

Issue 1: The PCT does not acknowledge or answer letter in a timely fashion.

You have stated that the PCT does not acknowledge or answer letters in a timely fashion and despite that fact that your letter were sent to the complaints manager, they were not treated as complaints, although you observe that it should have been self evident that they were complaints.

As a result of your outstanding concerns Mr. Luckie contacted the PCT who advised that they were in the process of reconfiguring to form part of Somerset Primary Care trust and that the consequent relocation of both staff and files may have caused a delay to some responses. In my reconsideration of this issue I have found evidence that the PCT has provided suitable apologies for the delays that have occurred and has also explained to you that they will not respond further in respect of those issues that have already been through their complaints process and on to the second and third stages of the NHS complaints procedure.

One issue in relation to the safe disposal of 'sharps' had been identified by the PCT as a new issue, but this had been treated as an enquiry and had not therefore been processed through their complaints procedure.

An examination of your email to the PCT on this subject reads as a request for information rather than as a complaint. Indeed, you specifically ask that the PCT, treat your 'enquiry' as urgent.

As such, I have decided that the handling of this issue of your complaint with the regulations that govern our work, namely the NHS (Complaints) Regs 2004 amended, and have decided to take no further action on this issue.

Issue 2 Explanation of the PCT's view that your son is not medically vulnerable and the handling of your complaint by the Healthcare Commission.

This issue has been investigated by the Health Service Ombudsman and is included in her report to you dated February 8th 2007. para. 16 and 30. It would not therefore be appropriate for the Healthcare Commission to consider this matter further.

Issue 3: Clarification of the PCT's position in relation to your son's application for Disability Living Allowance (DLA)

In his decision letter Mr. Luckie informed you that the benefits process is not an area that falls within the NHS complaints procedure and this issue was consequently outside the jurisdiction of the

ANDREW'S STORY

Healthcare Commission. In your letter of January 8th 2007, you refer to this point and comment that if indeed the benefits procedure falls outside the NHS, why did a doctor employed by the NHS have any opinion with regard to your son's DLA.

Ideally, a more detailed explanation of the role of the Healthcare Commission's complaints function may have been helpful to you in clarifying what we can and cannot investigate. The Healthcare Commission was created in April 2004 to improve healthcare. The Commission inspects healthcare service and provides information on our findings to the public and healthcare professionals. It is independent of the NHS and the complaints team has responsibility for reviewing formal complaints about NHS funded healthcare that have not been resolved by the relevant NHS organisation. Therefore, although complaints about, or dissatisfaction with the benefits system are not considered through the NHS complaints procedure, this does not preclude an NHS doctor from providing information to the Department of Work and Pensions (DWP) in relation to benefits applications.

If you have a query in relation to the benefits and services provided by the DWP, they can be contacted at www. dwp.gov.uk or via their enquiry line on telephone number 0800 882200.

Issue 4: Clarification regarding a reassessment of your son's vulnerability status.

You were informed in Mr. Luckie's decision letter that the further assessment of your son would have been against the criteria set down by Taunton Deane Borough Council and you questioned this statement asking where this information originated.

This information was provided to you in a letter dated September 19th 2005 from Mr. Colgan, Chief Executive of Taunton PCT, in which he states that 'the responsibility for decisions on any further application by Andrew for housing rests with the housing department and Taunton Deane Borough Council and he should approach directly to take up any review of his circumstances'.

Further more, in an email to you dated April 10th 2007. Mr. Brice (PCT) explains that it is not within the power or the authority of the PCT to make decisions on access to housing, as that rests with the local authority. Mr. Brice further informs you that Taunton Deane Borough Council has revised the process and they now seek independent advice on medial vulnerability.

It can be seen therefore, that the clarification you requested in relation to this issue had already been provided by the PCT in that both the Chief Executive and Mr. Brice had explained the situation and had provided advice on the way the new system operated.

Although I feel for the sake of completeness Mr. Luckie could have provided clearer clarification to you on this issue. It is evident from the above rational that the explanation you requested had already been provided to you by the trust and this would also have been evident to Mr. Luckie. As such, I have decided that the handling of this issue complied with the regulations and I have therefore decided to take no further action at this time.

Issue 5. Why the PAL's officer left the PCT.

As explained by Mr. Luckie in his decision letter, the reason why a member of staff leaves their post is not something that falls within the NHS complaints procedure and is outside the jurisdiction of the Healthcare Commission. I am therefore unable to comment on this issue further.

Issue 6: You state that you were told that there were no other complaints against the GP practice involved but there were five complaints on file and the GP had been through the Primary Care Trust's poor performance procedure. You state that you

were not told the truth by the Trust or by the Healthcare Commission.

Your concerns in relation to the performance of your son's GP practice were originally dealt with by the Healthcare Commission under another case number. Ms. Wray wrote to you on March 22nd 2005 with her decision. Ms Wray decided to take no further action on this issue because from the information provided to her, she was satisfied that at the time of your son's application the performance of the practice in question was not giving the PCT course for concern. The PCT therefore sought the opinion of the GP in accordance with their procedure for providing a medical opinion.

In her letter, Ms. Wray explained to you that the PCT had a procedure for the identification and support of doctors whose performance was giving cause for concern and this was in place at the time of your son's application. Ms Wray further observed that the PCT's procedure clearly identified the types of information which may highlight poor performance and these included complaints, PAL's contacts and a number of practice indicators, which the PCT routinely monitored through its Clinic Governance Directorate. Indeed, the concerns that you expressed were passed on to that department in accordance with the process.

ANDREW'S STORY

Ms Wray advised you that you had the right to raise your concerns with the Parliamentary and Health Service Ombudsman should you remain dissatisfied following her review. However, you subsequently included this issue in your later request for independent review dated October 28th 2006, stating that you believe information had been withheld from you and you were not told the truth by the PCT or the Healthcare Commission.

Although it can be seen that this issue had largely been dealt with in a previous independent review Mr. Luckie included this aspect of your complaint in his review, and in his decision letter he reiterated that the Healthcare Commission had been advised by the PCT that at the time you raised your complaint, there were no concerns about the performance of the GP concerned and that any action subsequently taken by the PCT was not taken as a result of your complaint. Mr. Luckie also stressed that information of that nature is confidential and not something that would be made available to a members of the public.

In reconsidering this aspect of your complaint I can confirm that I have decided that the handling of this issue of your complaint complied with the NHS 9 Compliants Regs. 2004 (as amended) and I have therefore decided to take no further action at this time. However, if you have a query in relation to a doctor's fitness to practice, you should contact the GMC who regulate doctors in the UK. The GMC can be contacted on the phone 0845 357 0022 or via their website www.gmc-uk.org

Issue 7 The PCT has failed to send a final version of the revised form as instructed by the Healthcare Commission

In his decision in this issue Mr. Luckie states, that according to the PCT's letter to Ms Wray dated August 15th 2005, a copy of the revised form was sent to you. Mr. Luckie advises that you should request a copy of the form from the Trust if you did not receive it at the time.

In your letter of outstanding concerns, you dispute this issue recommending that Mr. Luckie should 'read Ms Wray letter of the 9th August to Mr Colgan', as you 'only ever received an interim copy of the form and that was never submitted to Shelter'.

The issue of the delay to amending the form and the involvement of Shelter in this process has since been investigated by the Health Service Ombudsman and is included in her report to you dated February 8th 2007 para. 19 20 and 21, it would not therefore be appropriate for the

ANDREW'S STORY

Healthcare Commission to consider this matter further.

Conclusion

I appreciate that you might be disappointed with my decision to take no further action on the issues that I have addressed. However, I hope you feel that I have given careful consideration to the concerns you raised and that you found the explanations I have given helpful.

If you remain unhappy, you can complain to the Health Service Ombudsman about the substance of your complaints, the independent review and my reconsideration of this. I have enclosed a copy of their leaflet for your information.

Please do not hesitate to contact me if you have any queries or require further clarification.

Yours sincerely

Sheila Murphy
Case Manager Reconsideration Team.

A complaint to the General Medical Council regarding Now Medical bring the profession in to disrepute has not been resolved almost a year later.

ANDREW'S STORY

From Yvette Cooper to Jeremy Browne MP

13 April 2007

Dear Jeremy,

I am responding to your letter of 14 November to the Deputy Prime Minister on behalf of your constituent. That letter was passed to Anne McGuire, Parliamentary Under Secretary (Disable People) at the Department for Work and Pensions. Anne McGuire has copied to me her letter to you of 11 January.

The Government issues guidance to local authorities about the exercise of their functions in respect of people who are homeless or at risk homelessness. Under the homelessness legislation, local housing authorities must secure suitable accommodation for applicants who are eligible for assistance; unintentionally homeless and who fall within a priority need group. However, neither the legislation nor case law provides that applicants automatically have a priority need for accommodation if they have a disability recognised by the *Disability Discrimination Act 1995*. Nor does the Code of Guidance recommend that authorities should consider that such a disability will automatically mean that the applicant will have priority need. The Code states that for cases involving mental illness, learning or physical disability, housing authorities should have regard to any medical advice or social services advice obtained, but the final decision on the question of vulnerability will rest with the housing authority.

You have asked "who monitors the guidelines"? The Code of Guidance is issued to local authorities as guidance on how to interpret and exercise their homelessness powers and duties. Local authorities are legally obliged to have regard to the Code of Guidance. However, this does not mean that they must follow the guidance in every case. There may be instances where it would not be possible or sensible to follow the guidance.

The Courts effectively monitor adherence to the Code of Guidance. If an authority decided not to follow the guidance and was legally challenged on this basis, the authority would be expected to show that they had considered the guidance but had good reason for not following it in that particular case. If the Courts are not satisfied with the reasons put forward, they are likely to require the authority to reconsider its decisions or actions. The Secretary of State cannot intervene in individual cases and does not have the power to require local authorities to adhere to guidance issued.

ANDREW'S STORY

Where applicants are found to be homeless but not in priority need, the local authority must provide advice and assistance to help them find accommodation for themselves. My Department is encouraging authorities to take a more proactive approach to tackling homelessness and offer effective assistance, such as the provision of rent deposits, to ensure that any barriers to accessing accommodation can be overcome. We are working closely with local authorities and the voluntary sector, including providing funding of £200million over the three years to 2007/08 in the form of homelessness grants.

A copy of this letter goes to Anne McGuire.

pp Yvette Cooper

Minister for Housing and Planning at the

Department for Communities and Local Government

From Anne McGuire to Jeremy Browne MP

11 January 2007

Dear Jeremy,

As you may know, your letter of 14 November 2006 to John Prescott regarding a housing application was passed to this Department. I apologise for the resulting delay in replying.

I was sorry to read of the difficulties that Andrew has experienced. Although the Disability Discrimination Act 1995 does not cover housing and homelessness, I note that the local housing authority was advised that her son was not medically vulnerable so I hope it will help if I explain how disability is defined in the legislation.

The legislation does cover areas such as access to goods, services and facilities; employment; education; and transport. The Disability Rights Commission monitors its working in these areas and will, for example, take important test cases to court.

In order to qualify for protection against disability discrimination, an individual would need to meet the definition of a disabled person under the Disability Discrimination Act 1995, as amended. In general, someone is considered to be disabled for the purposes of the Act if they have a 'physical or mental impairment which has a substantial and long-term adverse effect on his ability to carry out normal day to day activities.'

However, special rules apply to certain impairments, such as progressive conditions, and some people are deemed to be disabled for the purposes of the Act. For example, since 5 December 2005, the Disability Discrimination Act 2005 has ensured that people with cancer, HIV and MS are protected effectively from the point of diagnoses.

The Act states that, for the purposes of deciding whether a person is disabled, a long-term effect of impairment is one which has lasted or is likely to last, at least 12 months; or is likely to last for the rest of the life of the person affected.

It also states that an impairment is only to be treated as affecting the person's ability to carry out normal day-to-day activities if it affects one of the following: mobility, manual dexterity, physical co-ordination, continence, ability to lift, carry or otherwise move everyday objects, speech, hearing or eyesight, memory or ability to concentrate, learn or understand, or perception of the risk of physical danger.

In addition, there are special provisions relating to the effect of treatment. The Act provides that where impairment is being treated or corrected, the impairment is to be treated as having the effect it would have without the measure in question.

In the case of a person with diabetes who takes insulin, for example, whether or not the effect of the impairment is substantial should be decided by reference to what the effects of that condition would be if the person was not taking the medication.

As I have said, the Act includes special provision for people who have a progressive condition. The impairment will be treated as having a substantial adverse effect upon their ability to carry out normal day-to-day activities before it actually does so, that is, from the moment that the condition first has some effect, provided that the effect of the impairment is likely to become substantial in the future.

Finally, as the policy issues surrounding housing and homelessness are the responsibility of the Department for Communities and Local Government I have arranged for our correspondence to be forwarded to colleagues at that Department for any comment they may wish to make.

ANDREW'S STORY

Best wishes,

Anne McGuire MP

Brenda Prentice

To Ms. McGuire MP   12th May 2007
Department of Works and Pensions (DWP)

Dear Mrs. Keane,

Thank you for your letter on behalf on Ms. McGuire and for a copy of the letter 11 January. It is the first time I have seen this letter. I can't imagine that Mr. Browne would not pass it on to me.

First let me tell you how my son does qualify under the Disability Discrimination Act. He has suffered from Hereditary Childhood Pancreatitis since he was 15 years old, (20 years). In 1999 he had surgery which removed his Pancreas completely. This means he has no natural insulin at all, and is a Brittle Diabetic. Without insulin he will die. He also does not have a digestive system, as the pancreas makes digestive enzymes; therefore he must take Creon, an artificial enzyme; otherwise he will die of malnutrition. He also has mal-absorption and chronic pain for which he takes prescribed morphine. Text books will tell you that Pancreatic pain is treated with the same pain killers as Cancer. The operation had a 50% of chance of rendering him pain free, but the operation failed. Morphine must be kept in a safe place as the law requires and insulin should be kept in a fridge. He also has serious depression and has been in a mental hospital.

ANDREW'S STORY

He does fit the criteria described by the DDA. He has 'physical **and** mental impairment which has a substantial and long-term adverse effect on his ability to carry out normal day to day activities'. He will not get better and will eventually die prematurely, a long slow painful death!

Should the Council have decided to take advice as to whether he is medically vulnerable to start with when the DDA say's diabetes is covered? The first homeless officer said my son would come under the national homeless legislation if he became homeless. When he did become homeless they changed their mind. The Local Government Ombudsman said that letter was written too long ago to be taken into account. (4 to 5 years, much of that time was taken up with the investigation)!

The problem is that the Council in assessing whether my son could 'live on the streets without detriment the same as any other homeless person', took advice from the PCT. The PCT said he was not medically vulnerable! So the Council would not help my son (not even with advice) they took the decision that he was not in priority need and they didn't need to house him. He could live on the streets.......

Shelter took this to court and the judge said, 'where advice is taken from someone with the qualification to give advice, the Council would be remiss not to take that advice'. He also said, 'Although I myself may have taken a different view, the council did have the right to make a decision! (He did not address the three points in law that Shelter wanted him to and refused an appeal). Council say they acted on advice from the PCT.

The PCT said, 'we didn't make the housing decision, the Council did, we are not to blame for their decision! Each blame the other!

The Local Government Ombudsman cannot look at a case that has been to court. They did look at peripheral issues and some changes were made by the council. For example, housing benefit is now paid and 3 years back pay was given! Not much good after you have lost your home!

The Healthcare Ombudsman said the PCT was only the messenger, the PCT asked the GP for an opinion, so it was not the PCT at fault, it was the GP. The GP has since been put through the poor performance procedure and has now taken early retirement on health grounds. The Ombudsman also said if the PCT had given an opinion, (they did) they would have been acting beyond their role. Was the GP acting beyond his role?

ANDREW'S STORY

During the investigations, the Healthcare Commission asked the ODPM for housing advice, they gave allocations advice, not homeless advice, but they did nothing wrong, as the advice they gave was not wrong, although it was not homeless advice it was allocations advice! On enquiry I was even told they are the same! I asked 'who monitors the guidelines' and after several years, eventually the answer is, 'no one!'

I asked the Department of Communities and Local Government to work with Taunton Deane to improve their housing performance, but they have refused, although they do have a 'team' within the department for doing that.

So, I ask Anne McGuire, what is to be done about this whole situation? It cannot be right for someone in my son's condition to be living on the streets. As a homeless person he would not even be able to sign on any doctor's register and would not be able to receive the medication required to keep him alive! Perhaps that is what officialdom wants?

It has been said that I am 'devastated that my son was not housed'. That is not right; I am devastated that any doctor could say he is not 'vulnerable', what sort of doctors are they? Specialist doctors should have been asked, as one said to me, "Just a look at his list of medication would tell anybody that he is vulnerable!"

Your comments would be welcome.

Yours sincerely

ANDREW'S STORY

From Department of Works and Pension. 23rd May 2007

Dear Madam,

Thank you for your letter 12th May. Unfortunately, although I appreciate your concerns and frustration regarding your son's housing difficulties, I am afraid I cannot help much further, since the replies you have had to date contained comprehensive explanations of this department's policy on the matter you have raised.

I understand that you have already been in contact with the Department for Communities and Local Government, but the issues you have raised fall within their remit and I have therefore forwarded a copy of your correspondence to them for further response.

Yours sincerely,

Brenda Prentice

Jeremy Browne
House of Commons
30th May 2007

Dear Brenda,

Thank you for your recent note. Having given this matter further consideration, the Ombudsman has stated the position clearly, and I do not think that any further intervention by me will make a difference. I know this is frustrating but, having written repeatedly to various authorities on this subject, I would not wish to create false expectations about what further could be achieved.

Yours sincerely,

Jeremy

ANDREW'S STORY

24th May

Lord Chancellor and Secretary of State for Justice

Dear Lord Falconer,

Please tell me why a Judge can refuse leave to appeal and why others do not refuse?

What can be done about a refusal?

Yours sincerely.

Brenda Prentice

Customer Service
Court Services   1st June 2007

Dear Madam,

Thank you for your letter, I am afraid that we cannot comment on a Judges decision, I can only suggest that you could seek independent legal advice from a solicitor as they maybe able to tell you the reason why the judge may have reached his decision once they have heard all the evidence

Regards.

Reply
I'm not asking you to comment on one judge's decision but as a general rule. What are the guidelines?

Yours etc.

Reply
As far as I know there are no guidelines.
Mr. Meek

Reply
Thank you, are you telling me there is no criteria laid down as to when an appeal is allowed and when it is not. I am talking in a general fashion and not in any particular case. Obviously a judge will refuse appeal when he does not want his

decision reconsidered; we all want to be right!
Does his need to be right, have no challenge?

Yours etc.

Reply 4th June

Thank you, I refer you to the Civil Procedure Rules
52.3 which explains when the courts are likely to
allow permission to appeal.

Mr. Meek

6th June

Mr. Meek,

I know what Rule 52.3 say's. But what I want to
know is on what grounds does a judge have a
right to refuse an appeal. He cannot know
whether rule 52.3 would apply at the time of the
court hearing. We would still be at the court and
he did not allow an appeal.

I'm asking on what grounds do judges allow
appeals and what grounds do they not allow
appeals? If you see what I mean? We hadn't got
to Rule 52.3 but some cases are given a right to
appeal at the time of the hearing at court. Our
judge said 'appeal denied'. He could not know
whether Rule 52.3 would fit or not. So why was
our request for an appeal refused, on what

grounds? I am asking a general question here, not anything to do with a particular case.

Yours etc.

Reply
We will endeavour to reply within 15 working days from today.

Further to the communication I have just sent to you I have just spoken to my colleague. We cannot tell you on what grounds the judge refused you leave to appeal. That is his decision. We can only suggest that you write to the judge asking for reasons for his refusal.
R. Meek

Reply
Thank you, but I was not asking in any particular case, but in general. There must be some guideline or something to say under what circumstances a request for an appeal is refused.

Yours etc.

Reply
As mentioned before this is laid out in the Civil Procedure Rules. How the judges interpret those rules is for them to decide. I am sorry I cannot help you any further.
R. Meek

ANDREW'S STORY

Reply
I can't understand why you tell me you will reply in 15 days and then say ask the judge why he refused leave to appeal. This is not a personal question I am asking you but a general one. Under what rule is any judge allowed to refuse leave to appeal?

Yours etc.

Reply 12th June

CPR 52.3 allows the court to give permission where the court considers the appeal would have a real prospect of success or there is some other compelling reason why the appeal should be heard. We can take it that the judge will refuse permission when he or she decides if and when this will not apply. I can only suggest that you seek legal advice as to the chances of success. I hope you find this helpful.
R. Meek

Reply
Thank you, but before we get to that stage, why can a judge refuse an appeal if he feels like it?

Yours etc.

Reply

The judge would have to give his reasons as to why he refused the appeal.
Kelly Tomlin

Reply
Well, he didn't, so what are the grounds he could do that on. Are we talking about just his opinion?

Yours etc.

Reply
I suggest you write to the court
Benny Stone

A reply from Taunton Court said Judge Cotterill retired about 2 years ago!

ANDREW'S STORY

28th. June 2007

Dr. Lynn Hayes
Parliamentary and Health Ombudsman
London

Dear Dr. Hayes,

Further to you letter to me 10th May I am sending some of my vast file and I request that these letters are looked at as a complaint to the Ombudsman, if it hasn't been done already. I have many more letters if you want them, I just don't know anymore what you want.

I am so confused by all the different case numbers and procedures that I don't know what is happening any more. As far as I am concerned it should all be looked at as one entity. It is all to do with the same complaint. As information has become known the case has got larger until I don't know which bit is being considered and which bit has to go back to the beginning again and start with a complaint to the PCT.

Enclosed is the Reconsideration by Sheila Murphy 29th May. She says in paragraph 7. Your letter was not treated as a complaint; I had asked for my enquiry to be treated as urgent, well, they never answered anyway! Again! Do I have to take this back to the PCT? Other issues have never been answered, that is why I asked again!!!!!

If the Ombudsman is right and the PCT were 'acting beyond their role' why has no action been taken over the other actions which must also have been beyond their role? There has been a lot of paper wasted on this issue and this is the first time I've been told 'the PCT acted beyond their role'. So what is to be done about it then?

DLA is not an area that falls within the NHS, so why did Dr. Morkane do what the council said he did? No one answers! What should I do about it?

Issue 4. The interpretation is not correct. Read what Mr. Colgan said, again. He said he would review Andrew's assessment and housing points. I asked how can the PCT have input to housing points. No one answers, again, why! It was the PCT who recommended the use of Nowmedical! No comment on that? Was that beyond their role'?

Issue 6. The PCT did not give correct information to the Healthcare Commission. There were 'concerns' over that Practice. See my remarks re Mr. and Mrs. Sylvester. The PCT said there were no concerns and yet they were monitoring the practice for 6 years! We were not told the truth. I included it as it had only just come to my

ANDREW'S STORY

knowledge. What was I supposed to do with information that had been withheld? The PCT didn't tell me, Mrs. Sylvester did! It is all part of the same complaint. Why hasn't anyone asked the PCT why they told the Healthcare Commission there were no concerns when there were? I know what the PCT told the Healthcare Commission, but it wasn't true! Mrs. Sylvester's complaint goes back a long way, in fact before this PCT. Dr. Harrison was fined £300 and the Practice monitored for six years! And the healthcare Commission was told, there are no concerns! I am a complainant, not a member of the public. Why will you take no action?

Issue 7. You will not consider this matter further. That's because I am right and you cannot demonstrate otherwise. There never was a final form and the PCT never contacted Shelter! I simply don't understand why no action is taken. The PCT did not do what they said they would. Had they have done so in the beginning, Andrew may not be in a mental home now! He would not have been caught by the inadequate form.

Sheila Murphy thinks I may be disappointed by her decision! I bet she is not a mother of a disabled young man.

As I say, this is all part of the same complaint and the method of breaking it down in the way it has been broken down by authority is expensive and time consuming and very confusing.

I think that's why it's done, so people like me get so confused that you hope we will go away and forget it. I will never forget that I came to you all for justice for Andrew.

Whatever the report say's, I am sure it will justify what all authority has done. The facts remain; Andrew cannot live on the streets without detriment! But you all say he can, if that isn't suffering hardship and injustice, what is? All the complaints I have made on behalf of Andrew should be considered together, not whittled down to pretend they don't matter. It seems that if it suits you all it is OK and if doesn't there is a way of getting out of responsibility.

Here is a poem by Andrew. The doctor say's he is now in a 'dissociate' state, Google that one! Driven mad by trauma induced by authority… and he is still self harming!

Too many secrets and too many lies
Too many unforgotten memories
Too many muffled cries
Too many words I wish I hadn't said
Too many nights of fear, anxiety and dread
Far easier to pretend and be okay

ANDREW'S STORY

For easier to let things slip away
Easier, yes of course why shouldn't it be?
But do I really know you?
Do you really know me?
Far easier to hide in the dark, far away
Safe from reality
Safe from the problem that won't go
away
I could scream and shout
People might look and people might stare
But ask yourself this
Would anyone really care!!!...

I hope those responsible are happy with themselves. The disease is enough to contend with without all blame he has had to endure. How can he live on the streets as homeless?

Yours in desperation,

PS. Do you really care?

Appendix 2

Stories from Stephen's PSN

New Member

I'm new here to this site. I'm John, 39, married, three kids (nine, nine and five), live near Wigan.

My medical history relating to acute & chronic Pancreatitis is quite short, just three years but I've been through the mill a few times with severe AP attacks, partial auto-digestion, six stone weight loss in six months and the almost obligatory lifestyle change associated with this condition.

I am currently healthier than I have been for a long time. I have what I guess so many people long for, pain free days and I'm actually putting weight on. I have CP with, the doctors say, about 80% necroses pancreatic tissue. The remaining 20% functional tissue does seem to serve me quite well at present.

So why have I joined the forum now, almost when I need it least...

I have witnessed this soul-destroying disease first hand. I have sat and watched my three kids drift away from me because I never played with them, couldn't talk to them because of the pain or was

ANDREW'S STORY

simply asleep during the day. I've seen the stress, worry and anguish of my wife, not knowing whether the next AP attack will kill me. I've watched my social life and friends abandon me and I've seen my promotional aspirations at work disappear because of my sickness record.

But I know I'm not a special case. I know most of you guys have gone through / going through all this so I thought that if I joined the group I may be able to offer help and support to people going through the sh** I've been through. If I can only help one person, one time in the next year, it will have been worthwhile. So, hello everyone, I'm pleased to be a member.

*

Hi John,

It's nice to hear your story and I am pleased that you are now pain free. I really hope that one day they can sort me out so that I can have some sort of life again. I have been off work since November 2005 with the illness and I am going back in April for my next check up to see what they say. I am not very optimistic as I am still only six and a half stone and not putting weight on very well still. I am still in a lot of pain (I suffer from CP) and am still to this day taking two types of morphine for the pain along with all the other drugs (paracetamol, diclofenac, multi vitamins and the list goes on). I live with my parents which is lucky really as they have been very good to me since my illness but I know that they still to this day worry about me and especially my weight. I have no social life whatsoever as I have been living abroad for seven years and lost most of my friends during that period and when I came back to the UK I started with this so the social life is still out the window at the moment.

I went to the docs yesterday and he says I have a chest infection on top of my other problems and he has put me on antibiotics. I still can't believe it has taken this long to get over this and that I have been off work for so long. I still wonder sometimes if I will ever get back to work. It is quite a stressful job but one that I enjoy as I help people to try to become debt free which is a very hard thing in this country at the moment.

Luckily I did not have any kids or anything when my marriage broke up. But I have just this week been to the Court for the final decision on my maintenance application, so it's taken nearly two years for my divorce to finalise. I always wanted kids but I can't see that happening now with my illness and my age (I am 41 in May).

Anyway, that's a bit about me, but thank you again for your story, you are an inspiration, maybe I will

ANDREW'S STORY

some day get back to work and a normal life like you. I really hope so, I would love to go for walks and days out etc but I am just still too ill at the moment.

Chris

*

Hi John

Welcome to the forum and it was really interesting to hear what you had to say about your experiences with Pancreatitis and how it has affected your relationships with family, work and friends.

It is very encouraging to learn that you are feeling healthier at the moment and that you have chosen to join the forum because you want to help others. That is wonderful. You sound like a very kind person.

I am 42, no kids, off work at present (I am employed by a children's charity) and very lucky to have a great partner who has helped me through this bout of illness. I was struck down by an AP attack caused by a trapped gallstone in late November 2006. I lost half a stone in a week but am eating fine now and building up strength. Just waiting to have my gallbladder removed in the near future. Like you I have good days and bad days. It is very difficult to be positive when you have recurring good health but I think that I am improving and my outlook is brightening. My main problem is that I hate being stuck indoors because I yearn to be outside. One of my hobbies is hiking (long-distance) so the illness has halted that!

Like Chris says, I do hope your children will understand as they get older why you were unable to play with them. My partner's daughter, aged eight, has just been off school with a nasty cold and I think being unwell has shown her how awful it is when you don't have your usual energy and she can appreciate why I have been laid up so much! She is a darling and ever so loving but she absolutely hated having a blocked nose and a cough and felt very sorry for herself!

Well, I hope you will find the forum useful, John, and a good source of true friends.

Kind regards.
Lindy

*

Hi John................Welcome to the PSN

I read through your posting and the replies to it

ANDREW'S STORY

and then left to visit some of the other threads running across the forum at the moment and I was struck by a great REALISATION! Your post had started off my train of thinking.

On this forum are lots and lots of people with the most horrific stories to tell, people who have suffered pain beyond the common person's comprehension of what pain is or can be, people who have faced death, people who have had their lives destroyed, people who have had their marriages destroyed, people who have had friendships destroyed, people who have lost their jobs and careers and even their faith in God.

Nowhere else is there such a large collection of people who should be depressed, hating the world and others, screaming out why me? Why does no-one understand what I am going through? People who could not really be blamed for having the most negative attitudes imaginable. People who should have learnt to hate as a result of the pain they are suffering.

But these people do not exist on this forum!

They may have a right to feel and have developed attitudes I have mentioned above - but they do not exist here.

Brenda Prentice

INSTEAD we have members with positive. outgoing and supportive attitudes

In the face of adversity, pain and personal disruptions we have all remained positive, seeking, giving and receiving advice and everyone of us in our own way prepared to face life, take our disease in our stride and move onwards.

I think I know now why this forum gives me so much pleasure.

Ray

*

Welcome John and thanks for sharing your story with us. I'm pleased you are feeling much healthier. We all have one key ingredient in common - the rare experience of many years of having not felt well; but remarkably we all remain positive and good humoured.

Ray's eloquent comments say it all about the members here and I certainly could not have expressed my experience with PSN nearly as well. In fact I think his words would be the ideal introduction page for new members. Thanks Ray.

*

ANDREW'S STORY

Welcome John to a brilliant site. Everyone here
has given me some great advice at a time when I
needed it. A few weeks ago I got very low and
didn't know what to do about my life. I didn't want
to end it but I didn't see the point in living. I live in
a very isolated place and do not work; the children
are grown up and moved many many miles away.
My husband although very supportive has a very
busy life so much that when he is home he is on
the computer doing more work. For me life could
no longer go on like this. Now thanks to everyone
on here (including Ray's wife] I have started to
turn things round. We are now going to move
house and area and start again. Although I would
love to move back to Yorkshire nearer to my
family we can't do that yet because of hubby's
work so we are looking at moving to a small town
part way there. That will put me in a better
position to get a bus or train any where I want. It
will be easier for family to get to and my husband
will be able to continue with his work.

All this as given me new hope. I am now sorting
through each room [one at a time] getting rid of
things we don't need and making the rooms better
for selling. I will be taking my time doing this as I
don't think the house will be going on the market
for some time. Part of our roof blew off in January
and we have only just got a cover on it. Not even
got an estimate for repairs yet as it's been too bad

for any one to come out to.

I hope by July we might be putting the for sale sign up, so if anyone wants to live on the top of a mountain with out standing views and lots of sheep let me know. In the mean time I am busy on the computer looking for my ideal home.

Best wishes for pain free days.

Margaret.

*

Great news Margaret!

Just sorting the rooms out will be therapeutic.

I'm not very good at that. I start then I'll be looking at stuff, reading things and usually put it all back again. You have to be really tough!

I'm not sure about living up a mountain - how do you get up there? I love the country but it has to be for holidays then I yearn for the streets of London. A small town seems ideal.

Anyway - happy house hunting. That's what they all do on daytime TV isn't it?

ANDREW'S STORY

Best Wishes,

Anne.

*

Hello John,
I hope this reply finds you ok, it was interesting to read what you'd posted about the effects on your children your illness has, when I had my long stay in hospital I didn't see my children (who were ten and five at the time) for the first six weeks of my thirteen week stay and I felt as though we had to get to know each other again, it must of been very scary for them to eventually see my in I.C.U with tubes/ tracheotomy etc, but they were brill!! But it's now eighteen months on that my son is sometimes very angry with me for what I must of put him through, my daughter on the other hand is very cuddly and talks about my illness quite openly (she always starts the subject) it's worrying sometimes, it's the what could of been that seems to effect both of them (and my husband and I occasionally)
Anyway a very big welcome to you take care

Sarah

*

Brenda Prentice

Hi Margaret

Nice to hear from you and it is wonderful to hear you sounding much happier and busier (too) with all the de-cluttering work. I hadn't realised you lived up a mountain and were so isolated so I hope you find somewhere nearer to civilisation and that will give you better transport links.

When we were little (I was seven and my sister was five) we lived on a very remote farm in Lancashire which was half a mile away from a tarmac road and my mum got terrible depression after my younger sister was born at home there, up in the wilds! Sometimes, loneliness and isolation are not such a good thing even though we lived in solitary splendour with the best views along the hills and valleys. No-one ever just drops in on you if you live in the middle of nowhere that is the problem!

Anyway, lots of luck with your house hunting. Hope you find exactly what you want.

*   *   *

ANDREW'S STORY

AP = alcoholics

I have just read through all the comments and
links and now everything has become clear....
although it was generally agreed that my first
attack of AP was caused by an ERCP, doctor after
doctor kept asking me about my alcohol
intake. Despite being told that because of allergic
reactions, I never drink spirits and only drink wine
or occasionally lager/beer shandy, the question
kept being repeated.

Being ignorant of the condition and in immense
pain, these questions started to really 'annoy' me,
to the point that when a new face popped into the
A&E cubicle, I shouted at them - 'No I do not drink
to excess!!' at which point they scuttled away.

I wear an allergy bracelet, maybe I should have I
AM NOT AN ALCOHOLIC added to it!! ☺

*

That's the way my girl. Keep your sense of
humour and give them hell. People do not seem
to believe what we go through until they have to
face it themselves.

Presenting at A&E because of the violence of a
pancreatic attack and being put on a bed "to sober
up" makes it very hard to keep a sense of

humour. My wife no longer takes any nonsense from any nurse or doctor - she tells them in no uncertain terms what they have to do and if they even try and mention alcohol now she reduces them to little heaps of quivering blubber. We had to learn the hard way though.

Best of luck and may you never have another attack.

By the way, "Just how much alcohol do you drink before an attack comes on??"

*   *   *

Weight Loss

Weight, that's a strange one!

I am 38 years old with CP, for as long as I can remember, I weigh ten stone give or take a few pounds. I used to eat like a horse and never put on weight, I loose pounds when a flare up happens as I can't manage food but I cannot gain any weight at all.

Some people say "lucky you" you will never be fat! But I say, please, let me put at least two stone on as I look far too skinny!

In reality, we with CP have enough going on

ANDREW'S STORY

without worrying about our weight! I bid you all a pain free day!

*

My twenty-one year old son, who has CP, is five feet ten and about nine stone. He has been up to nine and a half when he began to take Creon but when he has a flare up he can go down to six or seven stones (sorry, don't know the equivalent in kilos) You can literally see the weight drop off him and it is rapid too. My son is really self-conscious of his 'skinniness' especially when he goes to buy clothes and even the smaller sizes hang off him!

*

Hi my husband used to be twelve stone but since he had CP his weight is pretty bad, he must be about eight stone now, it's quite worrying as he looks really malnourished, his bones are sticking out. In fact he looks Anorexic, this really upsets the Children

* * *

GP's aren't always useless!

I'm going on holiday next week. I phoned the GP and asked him if he could do me a letter to explain why I'm carrying so much medication with me in case customs rifle through my bag and turf all the class A's out (oramorph / codeine / tramadol etc).

The girl on the desk said it would cost £10 for a formal letter. I thought well that's a small price to pay for an un-ruined holiday.

However, I had a voicemail on my phone this morning from the doctor saying forget the £10, if you have the attitude that you are going to drag your ravaged body half way across the world for a holiday, when he has to write fictitious letters for work dodgers and ne'er-do-wells on a daily basis, he's not going to charge me, his only Pancreatitis /chronic pain patient anything for the pleasure.

He said, have a great holiday, but make sure you put factor 50's on your scars!

I take back everything I've ever said about him; he's my new best friend!!!!

*

I am going to Mexico in a few weeks for a family wedding (touch wood) My GPs attitude is go as far and as often as you think your body will let you, enjoy every minute of it because you never know when these days will end.

ANDREW'S STORY

Yesterday I booked some private swimming lessons (frightened of going under water, but I can swim a bit) so that I can swim with the Dolphins

*

I think even if you can't swim, with our condition it is really beneficial to just let the water support you and lap around you, especially abroad it does you the world of good as you can just forget the pain and let the water support you. I've been known to be in the pool for three hours at a time. Doesn't do your skin much good but what the hey!

I am jealous as it's always been an ambition of mine to get close to dolphins. I once stroked a dolphin's nose as a child on a family holiday and I've wanted to do it again ever since.

Hope you have a good holiday, your GP has the right attitude!

PS, interesting dolphin fact - they are the only other mammal apart from us that have sex for pleasure. How can anyone know that? I mean have they asked the dolphins? "Hello Mr dolphin, I have just witnessed you having sex. Did you do it for pleasure alone or are you trying to procreate?"

Other sites

I have just copied what follows from an American Pancreatitis site.

'*I went to the University of Cincinnati today, and I have to say I was not impressed. The doctor first asked me if I was an alcoholic, I stated I was not, that I had never drank. He said he has never seen anyone who had Pancreatitis who was not an alcoholic. I have read much research that states there are a large percentage of people who have Pancreatitis for unknown causes/reasons; idiopathic.'*

Now does this not sound so familiar to all of us? Does it not indicate that most doctors need to educate themselves better on Pancreatitis or at least 'say nothing' about a condition they know nothing about.

*

Well said!

But, a point for us all to keep in mind - I read a paper on the web about three years ago that was about (acute) Pancreatitis cause statistics. It said that most general statistics on Pancreatitis that are published are American and that can be misleading to people from other countries. It said that the percentage of acute Pancreatitis occurrences due to alcohol (intolerance, alcoholism or whatever alcohol related activity) is HIGHER in the USA than other countries - 70% at least. It also said that in the UK and Australia that it is more likely to be 50-60%.

+*   *   *

SPECIALISTS

The thing is, although many hospitals have doctors and consultants that are considered specialists, unless you are lucky, they tend to simply be the most qualified in your particular hospital or area. In my experience, the knowledge gap between my local hospital (Which is considered extremely good in many fields) and the specialist I'm now seeing is immense. A great deal of information that my local consultant had given me has been completely contradicted by my specialist. I've been given pain control drugs that actually worsen my condition, been given the wrong dosage of Creon (CP sufferers staple medicine) and even had surgery that my new doc has said was completely unnecessary and actually harmful to me. I've also undergone two ERCP procedures that failed and gave me two AP attacks. My experience with my GP is many times worse. She doesn't actually know (and has admitted this fact to me) very much at all about chronic Pancreatitis.

The key is perseverance, dedication and being a right royal pain in the ass of your GP. Keep going to the GPs surgery complaining of your symptoms, keep asking questions he/she can't answer, keep insisting you need specialist help, ring consultant / doctors / secretaries who specialise in AP / CP to try and get them to see you and write letters to all

ANDREW'S STORY

of the above. It paid off for me. Remember, it's your health, your life and your quality of existence that is being eroded because of this condition. You have the right, like anyone else, to quality, effective care. It's just that sometimes it's damn hard to get it.

With regard to weight loss, it is a normal effect of Pancreatitis. Your digestive system cannot process food as effectively as it once did. Couple this with the fact that sufferers tend to lose appetite anyway, driven by the fear of pain if one eats anything. You actually receive a fraction of the calorific intake you once did. I lost six stone in a short space of time and once went without eating anything at all for eleven days - (Rather have malnutrition than the pain)

It is dependant on the severity of your condition but Pancreatitis can be controlled and managed with an effective drug regime, correct advice / information and some pretty stringent restrictions of diet, so don't be too fearful of the future. Just bust a gut to get on the list of a real specialist. I see Dr Makin at Manchester RI who's considered a leader in the field.

Keep in touch and Good luck

*   *   *

Brenda Prentice

I have some questions

Hello,

I started off with terrible pain and was rushed into hospital and thought to have had a heart attack. My second "heart attack" a couple of months later was actually diagnosed as Pancreatitis. That was in 2002. I suffered like you initially and had my gallbladder removed, but now, five years later, my pain is EITHER much less OR I have learnt to control it. I think it's a bit of both - many people with Pancreatitis are known to feel less pain as time goes by and also I can now tell from a range of symptoms when an attack is coming and I take painkillers straightaway. Once upon a time I used to wait to see how bad it got - not much point in that!

I eat pretty much what I want to eat but try not to have too much fat and take *Creon* with my food.

So you can feel better Carey. It will take a while, but hopefully you will suffer less and learn to cope with the pain as time goes by.
Anne.

*

ANDREW'S STORY

Anne,

You have really shed some light and given me a little hope. I really hope I am like you. I have been told a lot of things about this and a lot of it is very scary. It's quite overwhelming really. I am not sure what is more scary....the living in never ending pain with all kinds of complications and medications or the possibility of not surviving this. I know one thing for sure...I have never been one to let things get the best of me...

*   *   *

Just too young!

Just back from seeing my specialist!! I asked for stronger pain killers not allowed them because I'm not old enough!! So just because I'm under eighteen does it mean that I don't feel as much pain??! Still feeling very ill still blacking out with temp blindness and fuzziness what does she say but, "Don't worry this will go away you just have to put up with it for a while." I asked about getting my blood sugar tested to which I was told, no there is defiantly no need for that! You are not diabetic!!

Sorry for my ranting but I am in a well frustrated mood!!

thnx.

*

You must have a wonder doctor who can look at you and say, "You are not diabetic!" If I ever come to your neck of the woods, where-ever that may be, let me know who she is so I can avoid her!!!!!! When I first became diabetic I went to the local Diabetes Assoc monthly meeting I meet dozens of people I had known for ten to twenty years who were all diabetic and I did not know. I am not talking about Type Two people who just have to watch their diet but people like myself who inject themselves several times a day. They did not look like diabetics to me.

Sorry Robyn but blindness and fuzziness are symptoms of diabetes. I was watching TV News this evening and suddenly became aware of this fuzziness ..... I took a test and found I was 3.7 and this was only an hour after a large dinner. You may not be diabetic Robyn but testing is the only way to eliminate it ...... ask, NO, DEMAND, a laboratory blood test, ask for an HbA1c test to be carried out. RAY

*   *   *

Blistering Bosses!

ANDREW'S STORY

I've just come home from a visit with my dietician and she told me a most interesting story. She was in conversation with her original tutor who now holds the position of Chief Dietician in NZ. She explained the difficulty that I'm having in getting the correct supplementary food drink because as a CP sufferer I cannot stomach (pun intended) the fat based resource drinks. Chief Dietician, 'It's not a problem as Pancreatitis is only a temporary condition so no special arrangements need be made for the small time that they are affected'.

My dear sweet Dietician told her boss there was nothing temporary about my condition, I had been her patient for over six years now. Nothing more was gained from the meeting except that my Dietician came home to a blistering letter from her boss. In reply she sent a copy of Anne's poem.

The point of this is to say there are still people in senior positions that are totally ignorant of the nature of Pancreatitis or the impact that various foods can have on us.

*   *   *

Anne's poem

Brenda Prentice

Some people assume you are a drinker if you
have Pancreatitis.
Others, and particularly children, can't understand
why you don't want them to touch you - but it
HURTS!

If (for the Pancreatitis sufferer)

If you can keep your head when all about you
Are saying that you're ill because you drink.
If you can trust yourself when all men doubt you,
And not be undermined by what they think.
If you can wait and not grow tired of waiting
For ERCPs, stents and scans again,
And not grow tired of constantly explaining,
To others what's the cause of all the pain.

If you can cope with codeine and with morphine,
And PPI's and sickness pills galore.
And spend a goodly part of your life writhing
In blessed agony upon the floor.
Or curled up in a ball or sat in silence
And bending forward, leaning on a chair
And you can't travel far from public toilets
Because, Oh, you all know, I won't go there!

If you can cope with changing all your habits
Developed when your health was rather good,
And start to eat small meals and cut the fat out,
And always take your Creon with your food.
And give yourself erythema ab igne

ANDREW'S STORY

By cuddling something hot to quell the pain.
And you can't stand up straight because the
trying,
Has made you shout and double up again.

If friends can't touch you now because it hurts you
Even though they want to show they care.
And every task just leads you to exhaustion
With alien contractions you can't bear.
If once you might have had a drink on birthdays,
And anniversaries and special dates,
And Christmas time and now and then on
Sundays,
And now you can't go drinking with your mates.

If any or all that's familiar to you,
And you with iron will are struggling on,
Then pancreatic friends on here can help you,
It's very clear; you're one of us, my son!

Best Wishes

*   *   *

New Member

Finding this site some few minutes ago is, for me,
like tripping over a huge diamond when out for a
stroll ...... but of so much greater value! I have only
just started to look round here but feel at home
already.... if that is not being too presumptuous.

I'm from South Yorkshire and I am blessed with an unbelievably supportive and uncomplaining wife and three 'just grown' kids. My problems started many years ago with gallstone pain. They would not operate till I had lost a lot of weight ... so; of course nothing got done.... the pain subsided till I eventually forgot all about it.

Boxing day 2004 I was playing in a folk music session in a country pub when I got hit by the 'pancreas express train' and was carried almost unconscious out the pub, bundled into a friends car and rushed 20 miles to Dxxxxxxxx Royal Infirmary. I was at deaths door and was told if I had waited for an ambulance, I would most likely not have made it.

I had felt a bit off colour for a few days and it seems that a small stone had blocked the common duct and I guess the 'straw that broke the camels back' was all the 'goodies' on Christmas day. The poor old panc just gave up and burst.

Never get ill at Christmas/New year ... Patients in agony...Doctors in Barbados.

After initial suspicions of a heart attack, they did at least get the diagnosis right and shipped me off to Intensive Care where they stuffed me full of Morphine, Tramadol, Fentanoyl (and the lord knows what else) and starved me out. I was off my head and ranting for two weeks. It was a terrible experience trying to communicate to Docs & Nurses and them just ignoring what I said with that 'never mind him, he's off his head look'. They had inflated the balloon of the catheter in the urethra and seriously distended my prostate. They also had me laid flat out and I desperately needed to be sat upright.

Eventually in the wee small hours I ripped all the lines out and tried to get into the chair ..... The castors were not locked on so me and chair ended in a heap across the ward 😃 I fought the staff to get into the chair and refused point blank to be moved - what a relief that was !! Score one for freedom!

Fourteen days after admission, Consultant returned to find no scans had been done (or even ordered) and I demanded removal of the catheter ... which was followed by a bladder full of blood!

I had developed a pseudocyst which was then of manageable size but no treatment was forthcoming. Several attempts at ECRP triggering new attacks - all failed, the cyst grew and grew over the weeks and when they finally decided to drain it with a needle - it burst and flooded me internally - nearly died again. With the five litres they collected in the bag and the rest that sprayed all round the room the cyst was approx 6-7 litres in size. A fresh acute attack followed of course it was no surprise when I developed an infection and a deep seated abscess in the pancreas.

Finally I got myself transferred to another consultant, a personal friend who, thank God, referred me on to Professor Ali Majeed at the Hallamshire. The Prof had read my notes and promised me on that first day that he would personally conduct my treatment and see the job right through to the end. He was true to his every word.

What a relief to have a doctor who not only explained everything clearly and honestly, but who listened to every word I said. All that and a sense of Humour too 😃

It took best part of a month to get me fit enough to operate on, I was bright orange and some eight and a half stone lighter... but, nearly four months after admission, he successfully got the job done.

Thank you Prof - you are a true gentleman!

He did warn of the distinct possibility of developing a chronic condition and sadly a couple of years down the line I am on the long slow chronic slide that many folks here will know so well.

ANDREW'S STORY

Sorry to have gone on a bit, but it is a relief to be able to come somewhere that folks will really understand what I am talking about.

The terrible irony in this is that my best mate Pete, who saved my life that day and has been such a great support to me and my family since that day, has just been admitted to Weston Park with terminal Panc Cancer and is riddled with secondaries, sinking fast. Life is just not fair!

Stopping now... keyboard is filling up with salt water...

Dave

*

Hi Dave.

Before I welcome you I would have to know which team do you follow 😃 I've had P for nearly three years, eight acute attacks all hospitalisations, gallbladder removed, sphincterotomy, blah blah blah.

Currently investigating why I'm still in pain after GB removal. Pain comes and goes but there's no happy medium, it's either bad or good never in between and I have mammoth sleep problems. My specialist is Mr Charnley at the Freeman

Brenda Prentice

Hospital, Newcastle-Upon-Tyne. He too knows what he's doing (to put it mildly) and I agree with you it makes the difference.

I'm a bit worried about the future as well, I think we all are, but I won't let it beat me. We have to remember we have the disease, it doesn't have us.

Pringy

*

Thanks for your welcome

......."Hi Dave. Before I welcome you I would have to know which team do you follow".......

Only one team for me mate - The Pain Team! 😄
I had never realised just how common post Gall Bladder removal op problems were. Over 40% some reckon! Mine feels at times like it is still there complete with the 'hen's egg' it used to contain. Probably been replaced by the octopus arms of scar adhesions I certainly wonder if this might be a cause of a lot of my AP attacks.

I do hope they get topside of your problems soon.

I went to see my mate Pete yesterday; they let him out for the weekend. After 35 miles driving I got

ANDREW'S STORY

hit with a pretty lively AP 😊

I just made it the last couple of miles and the pair of us ended up smashed on morphine and sleeping, groaning and talking gibberish for the rest of the day before getting shipped home by my wife and one of the neighbours - Some sick visitor I am? Pete is holding up pretty well really and is slowly coming to terms with the dreadful reality. His bile duct is blocked totally and he is heavily jaundiced. He has got some scans today so they can try and sort out the nature of the blockage and decide whether they can attempt to stent it or clear it some other way so they can start chemo. Either way, secondaries are so advanced that I fear he will not have too much longer to suffer.

Thank you all for the welcome and your kind thoughts and encouragement

Regards

Dave

*

I can certainly relate to you and your wives experiences. I have found this site to be one massive source of help and comfort. Everyone on here is so positive in the face of this awful condition. My partner has just got home after spending six months in hospital...he had his pancreas removed on Dec 20th and was in intensive care for one month and the rest of the time learning to do everything again. We just got him home this week.... during the time he was in the hospital; I found this site a great source of comfort and help.

Keep smiling.

Mags x

*

Thanks for your story Dave. I have lived every sentence of it and can appreciate how you feel. I did laugh when you mentioned being treated for a heart attack - I knew I had Pancreatitis but on that particular occasion I was on a heart ward so when I had an attack I had to be treated for a heart attack which I did not have - thought that had only happened to me! I wrote about this "adventure" on another thread somewhere. I also recognise and enjoy your sense of humour Dave. "Patients in agony...Doctors in Barbados."

Bad news about your friend - I also have a friend who has just been told cancer is in his hip and throughout his body and all they can do for him is to see he does not suffer pain.

Anyway Dave welcome to this forum - I am sure it keeps me sane although my Aussie friends and

ANDREW'S STORY

perhaps a couple of the Poms would doubt the veracity of that statement.

Ray

*

You certainly do need a sense of humour when in hospital and a whole heap of patience for dealing with incompetent and poorly trained staff. Luckily, from the first to the last I have managed to hang on to both attributes.

I would love to prescribe a stiff dose of common sense to a lot of hospital staff... but it seems this particular drug has been discontinued through lack of demand.

During a totally botched needle drain attempt panic broke out and all antiseptic protocols went by the board as my pulse went way over 200 and blood pressure dropped literally below the scale. When eventually I came round again I immediately demanded to be put on preventative dose of antibiotic ... no way! So after 24 hours infection took hold and my temperature shot up to 104 deg F. The nurses kept taking my temperature with their magical 'in the ear jobbie' and despite all my efforts, insisted it was normal.

I am an old hand and always take my own

mercury thermometer in when I am admitted. I simply could not convince them I had a temperature and demanded to see a Doctor. Eventually some young thing arrived in the early hours and promptly stuck the same broken temp probe in my ear and pronounced me 'Normal'. Just to prove her point, she then stuck it in her own ear and got the same reading!
I remonstrated that a clinical thermometer can't lie and showed her. Unbelievable! It was the first time she had ever seen one and had not got a clue how to read it!!

I'm lying there in near delirium and sweating like a pig and she says I am normal! I finally grabbed her hand and stuck it on my forehead as I watched the look of realisation and horror come over her face. "My God - you are burning Up "!!

Where do they get these folks and just how do they get through the system to treat real patients?? It beats me. They must line em all up and give them a commonsensectomy as they enter med school

The upshot was that consultants appeared from nowhere and the hospital chief pharmacist was called from his bed at 3am to do some tests and mix a thermonuclear cocktail of antibiotics.

That day tested my sense of humour nearly to

breaking point and even now I struggle to find the funny side.

Keep smiling

Dave

*

HI Sarah,

You are quite right when you say a doctor can't know everything ...they are human so forget things and make mistakes. What frightens me is all those doctors that THINK they know everything, fob off serious questions with glib answers such as 'leave that to me - I'm the doctor here' and heaven help you if he finds out that you have actually read up about your illness or your medicines. Doctors with that attitude are in my mind downright dangerous to be near.

I am lucky in all the support I get from my wife who watches my back' for me pretty closely when I am really ill. I feel for those who have nobody to look out for them in hospital and have to just lie back and take it.

Dave

Brenda Prentice

*

When I had my first major AP attack I didn't have a clue what was causing the tremendous pain in my stomach, before I resorted to 999 call I tried all kinds of indigestion remedies thinking it was an upset stomach and I was so desperate to get rid of the pain I remembered that brandy can help calm your stomach so I had a large brandy. I arrived at A & E reeking of alcohol and of course the doctors assumed I was a heavy drinker, when in fact it was my first alcoholic drink for over a year. I got very little sympathy and in fact was treated very badly, I was left in a corridor for a very long time before I eventually got a doctor who very casually said, "You have Pancreatitis," he didn't explain anything to me and just walked away. I am sure that the smell of alcohol on me was the reason for his bad attitude.

*

The bedside manner of some doctors (trainees or fully qualified) is just appalling. They are supposed to be carers for the sick and suffering but, to be honest, some of them give the impression that they could not care less and your situation, Tony, just illustrates that. To diagnose a disease and then just leave you dangling is awful.

Some doctors could really do with refreshing their

ANDREW'S STORY

"people skills" on a course, if they ever had such skills to begin with! The ward rounds in the morning are terrible and you feel like you are getting a visit from the police or the Spanish Inquisition not a caring physician! 😁

Well, that's my moan for the day! Off to work now.

*

Hi everyone

Just thought that I would give a resume of my latest experiences in A & E with more pains, this time gallbladder related, in case it helps anybody who is going through something similar.

Well, I suffered in silence for about four days with bad back pain at about 2.00 am whilst I was trying to sleep. I rang NHS Direct and gave them a potted history and they said to just take two paracetamol and a glass of water and ring again if it got worse. The paracetamol did work for about four hours on that occasion and I just felt like I had been kicked really hard in the back, below the right and left rib cage. I was constantly needing to pass water (about every four hours at night) too, which is unusual for me.

Anyway, on Easter Monday night I got a kind of heart attack stabbing pain all across the front of both my ribs which was a bit scary so on Tuesday morning I went, reluctantly, to A & E at 10.00 am. By 1.30 pm I was admitted to the orthopaedic ward (broken bones), having been given an injection of pethidine.

The registrar could feel the gallstones in my gallbladder and he put my hand on them and I could detect them as well. The doctors said it was acute cholecystitis and the treatment was fifty hours of starvation and an IV drip. The antibiotics they gave me intravenously reacted badly with me and I turned red on my arm so they were taken off and I just had to rest.

I was given about four paracetamol for pain and a headache from hell (probably due to lack of food and caffeine) as I was only allowed sips of water. I was secretly hoping that they might be starving me for a reason, ie. to do an operation and remove the gallbladder but alas no I have to wait to see the consultant at the end of April and he will set a date. For some reason this time, they made me wear hideous surgical stockings for three days and have an injection in my stomach to stop my blood clotting. Never had this before and not sure it was totally necessary for someone my age!

Presumably my GB is inflamed/infected so I am on five days of antibiotics to try to return it to normal.

ANDREW'S STORY

On day three, dying of hunger but in less back pain and with fewer kidney problems, I sat in my chair by the bed, fully dressed, showered and looking alert, ready for the consultant's round at 10.00am and he asked if I was still in pain to which I replied "No" then he said "Do you want to go home?" and I exclaimed "Yes, please." The consultant agreed that I could go home and I felt 100% better. I got two pieces of toast at 10.30 am which tasted like nectar and the vomiting urge completely vanished!

Little information was forthcoming about what was wrong with me but my amylase was normal this time and I did not feel the pancreatic mid-back "alien" type, boring pain so I gather it was not Pancreatitis but cholecystitis. I kept vomiting green/yellow bile on day two, which tasted vile and it was impossible to get rid of the acid taste in the back of my mouth with just sips of water.

The average age of the ward occupants I was amidst this time was about 82 and the woman opposite me nearly died twice during the night due to water on the lungs and heart failure. The crash team, priest and her family were called in at 2.00 am both nights. Poor lady but she did pull through, thank goodness. Another 87 year old lady woke up at 5.30 am one morning and said to me, "What are you doing in my house?" and I had to summon the nurse to calm her down because she thought I was a burglar!

I am feeling quite disappointed that the hospital can't prioritise my GB removal and I will be quite furious if it perforates and causes septicaemia due to their inefficiency or another gallstone escapes and triggers AP again. What a saga!

So, another day, another episode of pain and dismay but I am hanging on in here to tell the tale and trying to stay positive.

Best wishes to everyone who has followed my story so far! I will keep you all posted. 😄 😄

Kind regards.

*

Holy crap, makes my ongoing "phantom gallbladder" pain seem inconsequential!

If it's any consolation I know exactly the type of pain you are describing, but I also agree with you I can't see why they can't prioritise it - it's a relatively simple op that only takes a couple of hours, and you are in tremendous pain.

Best of luck, keep us updated

ANDREW'S STORY

No Pancreas at all but still in pain.

I'm another one who has been through the total Pancreatectomy with little benefit. I had a partial Pancreatectomy (Begers) in 2001 followed by a TP in 2002. It's a familiar story. I was OK for a while but things have deteriorated over the last six to nine months. I am now taking oxycontin and oxynorm for pain and am awaiting a further scan at the Royal Liverpool.

The pain is grim and seems to be getting worse and since I've been on new pain killers it's thrown my Creon calculations all over the place with very unpleasant results.

*

My husband also had a total Pancreatectomy and also an auto islet transplant in January 1999 at the age of forty. As with your husband, my husband's life was probably prolonged, but at what cost?

He had been really really poorly for three years prior to his operation and was given the option of this procedure as if was a miracle cure. Unfortunately, this proved to be far from the case. For six months, he seemed slightly better. For the following year he seemed to be just as ill as before the op and for the following three years, he rapidly got even worse and spent most of the last year totally housebound and in continual agony. We unfortunately lost him in November age forty-five. Throughout the whole of this time we were told that his pain was 'healing pain' and that he would get better!

I know that for some, this operation is a god-send, but equally for others there is no improvement, or things get worse. I wish that all patients considering this operation could be given all the facts in complete honesty, in order that an informed decision could be made.

We are not guinea pigs for the medical profession to practise on and even animals would definitely not be allowed to suffer in this way.

*   *   *

Partners

I am the wife of someone who has had CP for some years. I read the discussion board at least once a week just in case someone comes up with something new... I don't see many on the board that live with someone with this awful problem. We don't have the pain, but we do have the stress and the worry, never knowing how they will be from day to day. Not knowing how to cope with

ANDREW'S STORY

them when they won't eat, don't sleep, our lives are turned upside down as well and we don't seem to be able to help. My husband say's just being there helps. I sometimes feel so useless and worry about what the future holds for him… Does anybody else who has a partner feel as I do?

*   *   *

Sleep

What I found most useful to get to sleep was to take my Sevredol tablet in bed when I was ready to sleep. I would lie on my back, swallow the pill without water (makes it/effects last longer), light off, breathe deeply to ride the pain, gradually feel my lips go numb (the morphine was starting to kick in) and then know nothing until I woke up in the morning.

Those peaceful pain free "sleeps" allowed me to maintain my sanity and fight the depression that you are only too aware of.

You can take Sevredol every hour if really necessary for the pain so don't be frightened of taking an extra tablet to give you a pain free sleep. **Just of interest**: the sevredol tablets can be broken in half for a half-strength dosage and a broken tablet still has a shelf life of 12 months. At one stage I was taking 25 mg of Sevredol (one pink and half of a blue) as my regular dose.

ALSO of interest: my pain doctor told me that you will never become addicted to morphine if you are taking the tablets for pain. The brain cells that control addiction and pain are the same cells. While working on the pain the same cells cannot be stimulated for addiction BUT lookout if you are not in pain!

We can't promise any light at the end of the tunnel but each and every one of us has developed our own "survival" techniques.

Best of luck

*

I picked up my calculator and did a little bit of computing. (I now realise that all I had to do was push the calculator button on my keyboard to have done the same thing - I'm just a little slow on the uptake)

ANYWAY - THE RESULT OF MY CALCULATIONS

I swallow over 9,000 pills a year

ANDREW'S STORY

I drink 86.5 litres of Medical Food Nutritional supplement

I inject myself with insulin 1,460 times a year

and none of this includes any injections or swallowing of tablets for pain relief. The above figures are just what I have to do to remain alive. Doing a little bit of calculation (using the calculator which pops up on the screen when you push the button) I estimate that I swallow almost another 1,**000 pills** a year fighting or keeping the pain under control. 800 of the pain control tablets would be Paradex tablets and the rest would be Sevredol (morphine) tablets of various strengths.

Quite frightening figures when you see them listed like that!

Ray

TAILPIECE: A computer beat me at chess once, but it was no match for me at kick boxing.

*   *   *

Brenda Prentice

Managing recurrent acute attacks.

I would emphasise from the start that I would intend any following discussion to be mainly with those folks who suffer and deal with recurrent acute attacks and have, through hard experience, developed a close knowledge of how such attacks affect their bodies and the best ways they have found to manage them.

To those who have less experience (may this remain ever so), I would emphasise that all acute attacks have the potential to be, or to become, life threatening and none more so than the first attack..... Always take medical advice and never take unnecessary risks.

Most here will know the usual procedure on admission or re-admission to hospital.

The wait to be seen, the lost notes, the apparent deafness of some staff to anything you tell them, the all elusive duty SHO the calls to his mates to find out what Pancreatitis actually is, and finally the token shot of the nearest painkiller to hand followed by yet another long wait to get onto a ward ...only to start the whole procedure all over again with someone else.

Multiply all the above by a factor of up to ten at weekends, and bank holidays and up to twenty for

ANDREW'S STORY

bonfire night and new years eve.

Standard procedure is then :

Nil by mouth...(food or water)
Saline drip
Naso-gastric tube
Catheter
Pain relief & blood tests

All you do then is lie back, starve it out, wait for the pain to subside, blood enzyme levels to reduce and, as someone hinted in another thread, the all important wait for that glorious (if a little stuttering) first trumpet to herald the return of life to the bowels.... yes indeed, our dear old friend the fart.

The principles behind the above treatment are all fine and aim towards putting the pancreas to sleep, giving it a good rest and then waking it gently from its slumbers, hopefully well refreshed and in a somewhat less stropy mood.

Now that I am better aware of the way acute attacks affect me personally, there are some aspects of the above 'standard' regime that do nothing to either refresh me or improve my temper.

Total abstinence from food is a given - no

problems there. If you decide to try and eat before you are truly ready, you deserve what is coming your way!

In an acute attack, my intestines effectively seize up and the continued flow of bile, having no place else to go, backs up into the stomach causing nausea and sickness. Apparently this is the same for most folks hence the N/G tube part of the standard regime.
The invasion of my stomach by an N/G tube always makes my situation worse. In addition to the minor but real moans about the discomfort and irritation of having such a tube fitted, there is the far more important fact that its very presence in the battle zone just seems to wind up my pancreas even more.

The build up of stomach acids, bile etc has to be got rid of and my own experience dictates that I need to expel the contents at intervals of anything from three to six hours. A couple of short painful retches and it is all over till next time.

I have had it written up in my notes that I will refuse an N/G tube. Any fluid input/output monitoring they need to do can be done just as efficiently by weighing the contents of the bowl. Likewise, I also refuse well intentioned offers of anti-emetics on the grounds that the body needs to get rid of and not retain all the gunk.

ANDREW'S STORY

A proviso of course is that if I get too ill to manage safely, a tube can be inserted.

I also demand to manage my own water input. Initially this is strictly swill out mouth and spit out into the bowl. Gradually I will retain small sips as nausea decreases and very slowly build this up. My own body is a good judge and soon tells me if I am taking things too fast as nausea, frequency and volume of vomiting increase. I always keep a record of what I drink and when and I generally surprise the doctors just how soon I can get levels and throughput up to the point of no longer needing IV fluids.

My other great bone of contention is the standard insistence that a catheter must be shoved in. I had horrific long term problems in the past due to incorrect placement and inflation of the retaining balloon and now strictly refuse a catheter in all but the most dire circumstances. Again, it is just as easy to monitor fluid output by weighing the contents of a bottle. One side effect of morphine is that it causes some contraction of the bladder valves and the urethra making it more difficult to pee and one side effect of Pancreatitis pain is that it is often hard or impossible to tell whether you need a pee or not. A degree of discipline and effort is thus involved to ensure the bladder does not get backed up and I make a strict point of trying very hard to pee every hour on the hour whilst awake and on waking after a sleep. Like everything else that happens to me in hospital, I keep a note in my little book of all attempts and successes. I have yet to encounter any problems with this method but am not daft and would readily give permission for a catheter should I run in to any problems.

I guess you have worked out by now that I take a practical interest in my treatments and may not always be the most biddable of patients. Doctors and Nurses at my usual hospital have however come to trust my judgement much more and I get less resistance on each visit. It is a sad fact that with our problems you often have to take a degree of charge in your treatment or you can easily come off second best.

I have dealt with many acute attacks at home.

A massive acute attack involving pancreas or cyst rupture is instantaneous and causes absolutely unmistakeable molten pain and is a 999 job or faster transport if available.

For anything less I find that with my recently earned 'Pancreatitis sufferer enhanced pain thresholds' this symptom is relatively easy to keep to manageable levels and my GP is understanding

ANDREW'S STORY

with morphine supplies.

Problems arise when vomiting and or lack of tolerance of water mean that oral morphine is not retained long enough to have effect or I begin to show the slightest early signs of dehydration. Either scenario is cause for me to bolt to the hospital for IV fluids and IV or sub cut. Morphine.

Well that is about it. If you are still reading I commend your powers of endurance. 😊

I would welcome all comments and discussion and I am particularly interested in hearing how others manage similar situations.

Please feel free to tell me I'm a cantankerous old prat for not conforming to the 'normal best practice' but a little explanation in support of your views, would be much appreciated.

Regards to all and.......

Power to the patient!

Dave

                     *

A very correct "wrap-up" Dave. Can't think of anything you have missed. My only comment is that I generally have been in too great a pain to take much interest or part in activities while a catheter has been inserted.

You touched on the wait before anything is done - A&E have your notes, they have (or have they?) listened to you or your care-giver that you are having a Pancreatitis attack but they want to explore every other medical condition known to man before they settle on the fact that you do have Pancreatitis and decide to treat it.

Ray
TAILPIECE:
☻ ☻ ☻ What is the definition of a "Will"??? - It's a dead give-away!

*

I would add, as I always do, for new readers or people who have just had their first attack.

People like Dave and myself know how to handle it at home and when to throw in the towel. If there is any miniscule of doubt, go to hospital.

Pringy

PS, catheters - I've had one inserted twice and couldn't see the point either. On one of those insertions they punctured my urethra, and the days that followed saw green pus coming out the

ANDREW'S STORY

end of my penis.

On the second insertion, some d...... nurse was making the bed and got her hand inside the gap between the tube and my bed and yep you've guessed it.......ouch

So I'm not a fan of catheters.

*

Ray!!

If I tried to recall and recount some of those conversations I have had in A&E I would, for sure spark another attack right here and now. Trust me though when I say, if I am conscious and able to speak at the time I certainly do not mince my words when confronted by such annoying little half qualified 'know-it-alls. ... Now look what you've done - you have gone and got me fired up again!! 😕

Pringy - I really do sympathise with your past experiences. There is no excuse whatsoever for such slapdash work and the consequences are both very nasty and long lasting.

Thanks for highlighting the dangers to newbies - Your point is most important and cannot be repeated often enough!!

Brenda Prentice

Regards

Dave

PS Pringy, I know the NHS are always hard up, but does your hospital really re-use catheters??? 😃 😃

*

All I can add really, is we do know our pain tolerance and procedure, I too as you know have experienced the inconsistent treatment from young wannabe's who have probably never seen a pancreas let alone know what it does and how to treat it. 😎

So, yes, power to the patient every time, insist you know what you're talking about because generally we do!!

😴 regards

Diane

*

Stupid comments re: alcohol

ANDREW'S STORY

I have a Google alert setup which scans all the forums in Google and tells me whenever the word "Pancreatitis" pops up. This got delivered today:

"Many people say alcoholism cannot be considered a disease because it is self-inflicted by poor behavioural choices and "a lack of will power." But are there not other diseases that are also caused by the similar factors? If we look at diseases such as certain cancers, heart disease, diabetes, obesity, gastritis, and Pancreatitis, to name some examples, we see these may be also a result of negative lifestyle choices. Many of these and other diseases are caused by overeating, poor choice of diet, smoking, excessive drinking, lack of exercise, or excessive stress".

 AND THIS WAS FROM A DOCTOR. So Pancreatitis is now a result of poor lifestyle choices! Amazing.....

*

THE DOCTOR SAID: Many of these and other diseases are caused by overeating, poor choice of diet, smoking, excessive drinking, lack of exercise, or excessive stress.

Hands up all the people on this forum who would like to have the doctor who said this about

Pancreatitis, to be our GP. "Now look here Ray, you are only suffering from these CP attacks because of your behavioural choices. Get some exercise man, change your diet and avoid stress and your CP should go away."

Thank goodness I actually attend a real doctor who understands Pancreatitis and if he is not sure he picks up the phone and rings a specialist and discusses my case with him as I sit in his office. My doctor generally rings to discuss medication.

Doctors having this attitude, it seems are quite widespread, and results in negative attitudes when we appear in an emergency departments.

Ray

TAILPIECE: Artificial intelligence usually beats real stupidity!

*

That makes me mad as well. The last time I went to the Emergency Room the doc asked me if I had been drinking as, "That is how a person gets CP". I haven't drank since I was told that this could possibly be CP and before that it was the odd glass of wine or beer on a hot day. I'm not saying I never drank to excess but since I had children it

ANDREW'S STORY

has been very rare! None of the docs I'm seeing have told me not to drink I have decided that on my own from reading about the CP.

*

I've noticed that it is so common to be labelled a drunk with this illness now that I try not to let it bother me anymore, otherwise it will just wind me up. Thankfully my G.P knows that I'm no drunk and my consultants know that I don't drink, but some doctors in A&E are an absolute joke. They spend so much time questioning me on alcohol to see if they can catch me out and discover that I'm a liar. Because I'm 28 and single they think that I must be out drinking every weekend like everyone else. It's this country's attitude to alcohol that winds me up the most though.

*   *   *

New Here

Hi,

I have been in this forum a whole eight days and already feel that I am at home and very much in the company of good friends. ☺
I came here initially hoping to find out more (in clinical terms) about CP and have found so much more than that.

Brenda Prentice

*

Welcome!
You will find a wealth of love, understanding,
knowledge and practical advice from fellow carers
and sufferers here. I very much hope your man
will come to realise that it would be good for him to
join you here too. Though folks here can't baby-sit
or collect kids from school, they can, I am sure,
through talking about their own experiences, help
you both to come to terms with, understand and
counter-attack, the ways in which this miserable
disease can disrupt relationships and lives.

Panc sufferers very often feel 'hard done by' and
that even those closest to us can't possibly
understand the pain involved but, men especially,
seem equally unable to recognise and understand
the effects that our illness has on our loved ones.

When I first got ill, I got to within an inch of my life
and simply don't remember much of what
happened in the first couple of weeks. I have
always enjoyed a rude good health and I most
certainly did not appreciate the gravity of the
situation. Being a fairly optimistic bloke, I think I
just assumed that I would get better no matter
what. My wife and family on the hand were
painfully aware from the very start that I might not
make it, indeed on two occasions, were told be

ANDREW'S STORY

prepared for the worst. They bore this burden, at the same time as shielding me from that knowledge with love and positive support.... and I continued to lie there blissfully unaware of all the grief they were carrying.

My wife and I have never had cross words in twenty five years of marriage nor did we when I was so ill, but I simply cannot believe how self centred I was and just how much I took her for granted. The crazy thing is that I could recognise this same thing in other patients and their families, and even commented on it to my wife! ... Talk about being in denial!

Likewise, my kids were always very caring and outwardly 'matter of fact' about everything. It was some weeks after I came out of hospital that I began to piece little things together and slowly came to realise just how bad it had been for all of them and how much support they themselves had needed from each other and their own close friends.

Unknown to all of us my twenty one year old daughter in particular had become very depressed and after professional counselling and every pill known to man, finally sought help from a forum called 'beatingthebeast.com'. I only found out by accident when she went to bed one night and left the page up on the computer. That sudden realisation struck me like a hammer. She lives most of the year away at uni and, though I knew she was a bit 'down' I had absolutely no idea whatsoever just how bad she was.

She felt she couldn't talk about it to family and it was the friendship and advice she found in that forum and the fact that she then had a safety valve to 'blow off steam' to folks who really understood, that did so much to get her right again.

I hope this little community will prove able to help you both through your trials.

*   *   *

Not again

Well it happened - I ended up in the Emergency Department yesterday - took about four hours of IV morphine to get the pain under control - at one point when my pain dropped from 9/10 to 5/10 for an hour, the pain at the base of the chest went berserk again back to 9/10 but the top up brought that back down fortunately. Interestingly my bloods were normal - a good thing but not without some frustration. It would be great to know what brought this all on, but that's just the mysteries of it I suppose.

ANDREW'S STORY

*

It seems that this symptom was on the rapid rise as I ended up in the ED on Friday night - morphine brought is under control after a few hours and now my burping is much less frequent and my chest pain is quite mild. So, I'm back to mainly abdominal 5/10 pain.

*

I'll share my frustration!

While that chest pain and classic centre of upper abdomen deep intense pain resolved down to about 2/10 since my ED visit on Friday - wow, someone turned up the dial.

Three times today I have been feeling "normal" when in seconds that centre upper abdomen pain hit me 7/10 like I was shot with a harpoon. It then began to rise and travel deep into my spine. It holds for about ten minutes. I am sure that the last time I ever felt that was at the beginning of my first two nasty AP attacks. Both brought on a feeling of nearly wanting to throw up.

Now it has resolved again - hopefully forever. Anyone remember that onset of pain?

Simon Aus.

*

I remember, Simon, I remember.

It's the unpredictability of this condition that I find the most annoying. You never know what's going to happen next.

Hope you are feeling better,

Anne

*

I remember the pain like it was yesterday.
Oh, it was.

Pringy

*   *   *

Is There a Cure?

Hi all,

I have a good old browse in your website and really need to ask....is there a cure for Pancreatitis acute or chronic or is this it? Constant controlled pain relief....

ANDREW'S STORY

My husband had severe pain nine years ago then he went for an operation and had all the cysts and part of his pancreas removed via Q.E liver unit in Birmingham. He was then totally pain free, until six months ago when he got a few niggles, this has increased and now we are told it will only get worse as his pancreas is calcified. Is there anyone out there who has been cured or am I asking for the moon???

*

Most of the people on this forum have Pancreatitis in one form or other, but it is very variable as to its severity and symptoms. Pain is one of the major problems, with most people it's constant, others the pain comes and goes, with perhaps weeks or months without pain and a few get no pain at all.

As yet there is no cure, just various methods of slowing down the damage and relieving the symptoms, although these are not always successful. So I'm sorry to say you are asking for the Moon, and I take no delight in saying that, sometimes in life we have to play our hand with the cards we are given.

Stuart

*

Brenda Prentice

Oh.................if only there was a cure!

Maybe, one day in the future successful transplants of the pancreas may become possible/routine. Unlike a kidney, which we have two of; we only have one pancreas, so someone has to expire to make one available.

Pancreatitis, in all forms has different reasons for attacking us, from alcohol to hereditary causes. It has different ways of trying to make our lives miserable, we learn to cope, and we learn to manage. We, on this forum anyway, have learnt to share our experiences and help each other as best we can. We all do what we can to prevent others going through the horrors we have been through. NO, THERE IS NO CURE, but GOOD MANAGEMENT allows us to generally live full lives in spite of the beast that dwells within us. Your husband was lucky having so long a "good spell" - I had a similar operation and my "holiday" only lasted twelve months. Sorry I could not be more cheerful but we on this forum "tell it like it is!'

Stuart summed it up well, "We have to learn to play the hand we were dealt with."

Printed in the United Kingdom by
Lightning Source UK Ltd., Milton Keynes
140511UK00001B/1/P